healthy eating for
pregnancy

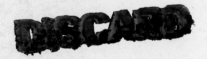

amanda grant

healthy eating for
pregnancy

the complete guide to a healthy diet
before, during, and after pregnancy

MITCHELL BEAZLEY

Healthy Eating for Pregnancy
by Amanda Grant

Healthy Eating for Pregnancy is meant to be used as a general reference and recipe book. While the author believes the information and recipes it contains are beneficial to health, the book is in no way intended to replace medical advice. You are therefore urged to consult your health-care professional about specific medical issues or complaints.

First published in Great Britain in 2001 by Mitchell Beazley, an imprint of Octopus Publishing Group Limited, 2–4 Heron Quays, London E14 4JP.

Reprinted 2002, 2008

Distributed in the United States and Canada by Sterling Publishing Co. Inc., 387 Park Avenue South, New York, NY 10016-8810

A CIP catalogue record for this book is available from the British Library.

ISBN 978 1 84533 421 5

While all reasonable care has been taken during the preparation of this edition, neither the publisher, editors, nor the authors can accept responsibility for any consequences arising from the use thereof or from the information contained therein.

Commissioning Editor: Rebecca Spry
Executive Art Editor: Phil Ormerod
Managing Editor: Emma Rice
Design: Miranda Harvey
Editors: Jo Richardson, Jamie Ambrose
Counsultant Nutritionist: Tanya Carr
Production: Jessame Emms
Index: John Noble
Photography: William Reavell

Typeset in Helvetica Neue
Printed and bound by Toppan Printing Company in China

contents

these symbols are used in the recipe section:

suitable for freezing

suitable for toddlers

prepare in advance

preconception diet

preconception
care

At conception, if both parents have paid similar care and attention to their health, they are more likely to produce a healthy baby.

preparing for pregnancy

In order to create a healthy baby, why not consider applying the principles used in organic farming?

Organic farmers prepare the soil with natural nutrients over many years and avoid processed chemicals. This results in strong, vigorous, healthy plants which are able to resist diseases and pests. All the vitamins, minerals, enzymes, and essential nutrients are in balance.

At conception, if both parents have paid similar care and attention to their health, they are more likely to produce a healthy baby.

Preconception care is the term given to the method of bringing both parents as close to optimum health as possible *before* they try to conceive. It creates the healthiest physical environment for a growing embryo.

Preconception care has the benefit of maximizing the chances of a healthy sperm, ova, and uterus; in turn, this helps to foster a healthy pregnancy.

history of preconception care

Preconception care has been around for many centuries—there are even references to it in the Bible: "And the angel of the Lord appeared unto the woman, and said unto her: '...thou shalt conceive, and bear a son. Now therefore beware, I pray thee, and drink not wine nor strong drink, and eat not any unclean thing.'" (Ref. 1.1)

Thousands of much-wanted babies are stillborn or miscarried each year, and many are born frail, often as a result of a lack of information about preconception care. Foresight's objective is to pass on this knowledge to help all parents achieve a healthy, full-term pregnancy. Some experts believe that it is possible to reduce, and in many cases, eliminate, infertility, pregnancy, and birth problems.

conception problems

It is often too late to prevent many problems once a woman knows that she is pregnant.

Alcohol and smoking are at their most hazardous during the earliest stages of pregnancy, when cell division is at its highest. It is therefore important that if a woman decides to become pregnant, she should avoid these substances from the first opportunity. Having said that, if you discover you are already pregnant, it is obviously still advisable to stop smoking and drinking as soon as possible.

Approximately one in six couples will have some difficulty conceiving. About one in 10 couples will take more than a year to conceive and one in 20 more than two years. Even in the most fertile couples, the chance of becoming pregnant in each menstrual cycle is only 25 per cent (Ref. 1.2).

In order to prepare fully for conception, the issues in the following pages need to be considered.

preconception nutrition

...it is advised by experts that couples start putting good nutrition into practice at least four months—the longer, the better—before trying to conceive.

"We are what we eat," as the saying goes. We need top-quality "fuel" in order for our bodies to function properly and to produce healthy eggs or sperm. In other words, good nutrition is essential for good health.

The food we eat has an impact on every cell in our bodies. Eating healthily can help women to conceive and give birth to a healthy baby—see pages 34–61 for more information about healthy eating.

Good nutrition for men helps ensure healthy sperm and sexual activity. Poor nutrition in women can lead to fertility problems as highlighted by birth-rate studies during famines (Ref. 1.3).

In fact, the inability to reproduce can be one of the first signs of imperfect nutrition. This vital link between nutrition and fetal development has been researched by a number of scientists. The work of Isobel Jennings, Weston Price, E J Underwood, Donald Oberleas, Donald Caldwell, Lucille Hurley, Bert Vallee, and many others has drawn attention to the role played by a lack of nutrients in reproductive problems under experimental conditions.

Such studies have found that, in many cases, almost all the commonly seen birth defects can be reduced or eliminated by changing the diet .

It is advised by experts that couples start putting good nutrition into practice at least four months— the longer, the better—before trying to conceive. This will at least give the body a chance to correct any nutritional deficiencies. This four-month "minimum" period is also recommended because it takes at least three months for men to produce a new batch of sperm and women's eggs to mature, ready for ovulation.

You might like to ask your doctor to refer you to a state-registered dietician or registered nutritionist, specializing in diet for preconception and pregnancy. He or she will be able to assess your nutrient intake as well as point out any signs of nutrient deficiencies, and advise appropriate action.

At the end of the four months, the assessment should be repeated. You will then be given a maintenance program to adhere to until you conceive and ideally for life! (Ref. 1.4).

A well-balanced vegetarian diet is extremely healthy for all life stages, including preconception and pregnancy...

vegetarian & vegan

A well-balanced vegetarian diet can provide the nutritional and calorific requirements for fertility. A poorly planned vegetarian diet, just like a poorly planned diet that includes meat, can result in decreased fertility (*Ref. 1.5*).

Vegans may take longer to conceive, according to *Nutrition and Pregnancy: A Complete Guide from Preconception to Post-delivery* by Judith E Brown (*Ref. 1.6*). The author found that, while vegans do not tend to be infertile, they may take longer to conceive because a high-plant diet appears to increase menstrual cycle length, causing less frequent ovulation. This is no cause for concern, however; it is simply something for vegans to keep in mind when trying to conceive.

organic

There is a growing awareness of the benefits of eating organic food. For instance, research carried out in 1994 by the Department of Occupational Medicine in Denmark found that men who regularly ate organic food had twice the sperm count of those on a conventional diet. It is probably just a matter of time before the health benefits of organic foods are proven scientifically.

fertility: what to eat

fats

Contrary to popular belief, not all fats are bad. However, before reaching for the chocolates or the cherry cheesecake lurking menacingly in the back of the fridge, it is worth bearing in mind that most of us eat too much of the wrong types of fat and not enough of the beneficial kind. Some of the "good" types of fats are known as "essential" fats, while those generally considered "bad" are known as "saturated fats." Chocolate and cream are in the "bad" category!

There are two fatty acids that the body cannot make; they must be sourced from what we eat.

essential fats

Fat is made up of substances called fatty acids. There are two fatty acids that the body cannot make; they must be sourced from what we eat. Known as essential (polyunsaturated) fatty acids (EFAs) (*see* page 44 for more details) these are called alpha-linolenic acid and linoleic acid. They are vital for good health.

We need EFAs to keep the body warm, the skin and arteries supple, and the hormones in balance. In fact, they have a significant effect on every system in the body, including reproduction.

From EFAs we produce beneficial substances called prostaglandins, which behave as hormones. If these become imbalanced, it may be difficult to conceive. However, this situation may be rectified in some people by increasing good sources of essential fats in the diet.

Also, sperm is rich in prostaglandins, which is why men will benefit from essential fats in the diet. Semen taken from poor sperm samples has been found to lack an adequate amount of these beneficial prostaglandins (*Ref 1.7*).

Essential fats are found in oils, oily fish, nuts, and seeds. It is possible to maintain an acceptable daily intake of essential fatty acids by eating a handful of seeds and nuts, or by using good-quality oils in cooking and dressings. It is also advisable to include oily fish such as mackerel and sardines in our diet.

saturated fats

Even though they stimulate estrogen, saturated fats can adversely affect fertility. A diet high in saturated fats can also restrict the usage of the EFAs in the body.

Saturated fats tend to be mainly solid at room temperature. They are primarily sourced from animals, so you may need to restrict your intake of foods like dairy produce (including butter, eggs, whole milk, yogurt, and cheese) and meats.

fiber

It has been found that a healthy, high-fiber diet will reduce high levels of toxic metals, such as lead.

An adequate supply of fiber in the diet helps the human body to achieve three main objectives.

It ensures that nutrients are absorbed in a systematic, steady fashion, and helps to produce substances that fight against "free-radical" damage (free radicals are naturally occurring oxygen molecules that damage human and animal tissue and are thought to play a key role in the aging process).

In addition, fiber keeps the bowels healthy and prevents constipation. This is particularly important for fertility because women need to get rid of chemicals, pesticides, heavy toxic metals, and other toxins that may have an adverse affect on their reproductive systems. It has been found that a healthy, high-fiber diet can help reduce high levels of toxic metals, such as lead.(Ref. 1.9).

Women also need to excrete old estrogens (female hormones) from their bodies in order to help keep their reproductive systems in optimum balance. Fiber contained in whole grains and fruit and vegetables enables the body to do this.

To increase fiber intake, eat plenty of fresh fruit, vegetables (whenever possible raw, but also cooked), whole grains (brown rice, whole-wheat bread, oats, whole-grain crackers, whole-wheat pasta, etc.), beans, nuts, and seeds.

carbohydrates

It is advisable
to eat as
many complex
carbohydrates
as possible and
as few simple
carbohydrates
as possible.

Like fats, carbohydrates provide the body with energy. There are two types of carbohydrates: simple and complex. Simple carbohydrates (sugars) are found in foods such as cakes, cookies, and jams, as well as honey. Complex carbohydrates are found in whole-grain foods and whole-wheat flours. Good examples include whole-wheat pasta, brown rice, and potatoes.

It is advisable to eat as many complex carbohydrates as possible and as few simple carbohydrates as possible. There are a few reasons for this: simple carbohydrates are often found in foods high in sugars and fats but containing very little else. Consequently, these foods are not very nutrient dense. If your diet relies heavily on these foods, you may run the risk of not having a sufficient supply of all the essential nutrients.

Also, if eaten on their own, simple carbohydrates can cause blood-sugar levels to fluctuate, which is best avoided as this may affect hormonal cycles. If you do eat simple carbohydrates, it is advisable to combine them with the complex variety to reduce any blood-sugar swings. Better still, aim to avoid sugar or sugar-based snacks altogether.

protein

A low intake of protein can reduce chances of conception, so women must make sure that they eat a good range of high-quality protein foods. As most of us gain much of our required protein from meat and dairy products, vegetarians—and vegans even more so—need to pay particular attention to this aspect of their diet. For more information about protein and good vegetarian sources of protein, *see* page 47.

zinc

Zinc is important to the body for a number of reasons. It helps growth, aids healing, assists in coping with stress, promotes a healthy brain and nervous system—particularly in a growing fetus—helps ensure that energy supplies are both stable and sustained, and boosts our ability to maintain a healthy immune system.

Much research has been carried out on zinc and its effects on the human body. There is a fair weight of evidence to suggest that it is important for fertility in both men and women.

...research has been carried out on zinc and its effects on the human body. There is a fair weight of evidence to suggest that it is important for fertility in both men and women.

males

The main conclusions of the numerous studies carried out on zinc and male fertility are that zinc is needed for the proper development of sperm (*Ref 1.8*). In addition, if there is a lack of zinc, the sperm may not be able to penetrate the egg (*Ref 1.9*). Zinc is also necessary for the production of the reproductive hormones estrogen and progesterone (*Ref 1.10*). Finally, zinc plays a vital role in cell division.

females

As far as the effects of zinc on the female reproductive system are concerned, the Foresight Association has found that many women having difficulty conceiving show high levels of copper and low levels of zinc. It has also been found that the contraceptive pill can inhibit the absorption of zinc. In addition, if levels of zinc are not at an optimum, conception is difficult; there are also risks that any babies which are conceived may have a low birth weight and other possible complications (*Ref 1.11*).

As a result of these issues, it is important to ensure that adequate levels of zinc are present in the diet both before and at the time of conception.

Zinc levels can be improved by eating zinc-rich foods. Such sources include lamb, turkey, sardines, hard cheeses, wheat germ, and whole-grain cereals, legumes such as lentils, beans, and chickpeas, green vegetables such as watercress, spinach, and peas, and fruits such as dried apricots and figs.

...if levels of zinc are not at an optimum, conception is difficult; there are also risks that any babies which are conceived may have a low birth weight and other possible complications.

manganese

Like zinc, manganese is needed to help prevent infertility in both men and women. The body also uses it to help control blood-sugar levels and assist with cell protection and the formation of bones, skin, and cartilage.

Low manganese levels have also been linked to decreased libido in both sexes. In addition, babies born to mothers with low manganese levels may be more prone to birth defects.

A well-balanced diet is likely to provide sufficient manganese. Good specific sources of it include tropical fruits, nuts, seeds, and whole grains.

selenium

Good levels of selenium are also essential for the healthy development of sperm. Blood-selenium levels have been found to be lower in men with low sperm counts.

Selenium is an antioxidant—a group of substances believed to reduce the risk of cancer, heart disease, and other age-related diseases.

Selenium can also help to prevent birth defects and miscarriages. It can help protect against poisoning from heavy toxic metals (see pages 26-7 and 30).

Good levels of selenium are also essential for the healthy development of sperm. Blood-selenium levels have been found to be lower in men with low sperm counts (Ref 1.12).

Selenium is found in nuts such as Brazil nuts; seeds such as sunflower seeds; milk; whole-wheat bread (but only if made with flour grown in selenium-rich soil), cheese, eggs, chicken, shellfish, and fish.

folic acid

There are a number of reasons why women need folic acid in their diets. First of all, it helps to create healthy blood cells; insufficient supplies can result in anemia. Secondly, it helps the body absorb iron.

Folic acid is also needed in the production of genetic material. It is important in fertility as well as during pregnancy, and it can help to prevent spina bifida (see page 56).

The human body cannot store large quantities of folic acid; in fact, we can only store a supply that is sufficient for a maximum of two or three months. It is therefore important to eat foods rich in folic acid as part of the daily diet.

Good sources of folic acid include green, leafy vegetables; asparagus; oranges; and wheat germ. However, the content of folic acid in food tends to reduce over time; the longer they are left after picking, the lower the folic acid content. We need to eat foods as fresh as possible and keep cooking times as short as possible in order to gain the maximum benefit from the nutritional value of these foods. Salads, stir-fries, and steamed vegetables are all great ways of enjoying vegetables rich in folic acid.

The contraceptive pill and other forms of medication (aspirin and indigestion remedies) as well as alcohol may decrease the amount of folic acid stored in the body.

In addition to eating foods rich in folic acid, the US Food and Drug Administration recommends that women of childbearing age should include 400 micrograms (mcg) of folic acid in their diet every day. Source: TimeLife Drug and Natural Medicine Advisor (Virginia, 1997).

The human body cannot store large quantities of folic acid; in fact, we can only store a supply that is sufficient for a maximum of two or three months.

B$_{12}$

Vitamin B$_{12}$ has many roles to play in general well-being. It is required to develop and maintain a healthy nervous system. We need it to help with the digestion of food and the conversion of food into energy. It is also necessary to produce red blood cells.

Lack of this vitamin may result in a form of anemia which is associated with infertility. Low levels of B$_{12}$ can also contribute toward a low sperm count. Studies have demonstrated the potential of vitamin B$_{12}$ for increasing male fertility (*Ref 1.13*).

Women in particular need to make sure that their diets are rich in vitamin B$_{12}$. Good sources are primarily of animal origin, including milk and cheese. Other foods include oily fish such as sardines. Vegans need to pay particular attention to their intake of B$_{12}$.

B$_6$ (pyridoxine)

We need vitamin B$_6$ to help convert protein into energy and aid with the functioning of both the nervous and immune systems.

Women who have trouble conceiving have been known to benefit from increasing their intake of vitamin B$_6$. In some women, B$_6$ has been shown to increase levels of progesterone, a female hormone needed to maintain a healthy womb lining and to support growth of a fertilized egg (*Ref. 1.14*).

The best way to increase your vitamin B$_6$ levels is to eat vitamin B$_6$-rich foods. These include dark green leafy vegetables, nuts, lentils, peanuts, bananas, and melons.

Women who have trouble conceiving have been known to benefit from increasing their intake of vitamin B$_6$.

vitamin c

Vitamin C, a powerful antioxidant, is needed for growth and health of body tissue, and it is necessary for the healing of wounds. It can also protect the sperm and its DNA from damage (*Ref 1.15*). Studies have shown how male fertility has been improved when men increase their vitamin C intake (*Ref 1.16*). When sperm enter a woman's body, antibodies directed against them cause the sperm to clump together, which renders them less likely to fertilize the egg. Vitamin C helps to reduce this process of agglutination.

Vitamin C is a water-soluble vitamin that cannot be stored in the body in large amounts. If we consume too much, our bodies will just get rid of it. We rely on our diet for vitamin C, unlike nearly all other animals who are able to make the vitamin themselves. Fruits and vegetables are the main sources of this vitamin. If we eat five servings of fresh fruits and vegetables a day, we should be eating enough to get our daily requirement. Particularly good fruits include strawberries, oranges, kiwi fruit, black currants, mangoes, papayas, lychees, and peaches. Good vegetable sources include red peppers, spinach, watercress, and peas.

vitamin A

As well as being necessary for growth, healthy skin, hair, and vision, vitamin A is essential for reproduction. It maintains healthy tissues that line all external and internal surfaces of the body, including the linings of the vagina and uterus. During pregnancy, it is also needed by the developing baby.

It is therefore important that, both before and after conception, women receive a good intake of vitamin A. If you eat a well-balanced diet, you should receive enough vitamin A from your food. Good animal sources include milk, cheese, and egg yolks.

Betacarotene, a substance found in orange, yellow, and green vegetables, is converted into vitamin A in the body.

Vitamin A maintains healthy tissues that line all the external and internal surfaces of the body.

iron

We need iron for healthy blood and muscles. Iron is also known to have helped women with infertility problems.

We need iron for healthy blood and muscles. Iron is also known to have helped women with infertility problems (*Ref 1.17*). It is therefore advisable to include iron-rich foods in your daily diet.

Good sources of iron include lean meat, eggs (during pregnancy, make sure that these are thoroughly cooked), and green leafy vegetables such as spinach and broccoli. Iron in non-meat foods is not as easily absorbed by the body, so we need to eat more of these foods to gain the equivalent amount of iron.

Vitamin C aids in the absorption of iron, so it is also advisable to eat a good supply of foods rich in this vitamin at the same time.

Drinks such as tea and coffee contain tannins, which can inhibit the absorption of iron, so it is advisable to keep these drinks to an absolute minimum. This is sensible advice for good general health as well. See page 28 for information about caffeine and fertility.

vitamin E

Vitamin E has been shown to be of benefit to both male and female fertility.

Like vitamins C and A, vitamin E is a powerful antioxidant. These substances have the ability to fight free radicals linked to cancer, coronary heart disease, and infertility, which destroy cells and can speed up the aging process.

Vitamin E has been shown to be of benefit to both male and female fertility and is of particular importance for those over 35. It is also necessary for the production of healthy sperm and, along with zinc, manganese, and vitamin B_{12}, is vital for a good sperm count. Vitamin E is also needed for the development and maintenance of strong cells, particularly in the blood.

It is therefore a good idea to make sure that your diet contains a plentiful supply of vitamin E and other antioxidant vitamins. It is possible to receive adequate amounts of vitamin E from a well-balanced diet that includes such foods as mangoes, sweet potatoes, watercress, avocados, spinach, and vegetable oils such as olive oil.

organic foods

There is also a school of thought that believes organic food may be better nutritionally, but this is still being researched.

Some experts believe that eating an organic whole-food diet will help improve fertility. Some research is based on the work carried out by the Foresight Association (*see* "Useful addresses" page 143). Foresight has helped thousands of people to conceive healthy babies, including those who have failed IVF.

Part of the Foresight program is based on eating a healthy, well-balanced diet composed of as much organic food as possible. Just like many experts, the Foresight organization states that it is better to eat organic foods that are free from pesticide residues than their non-organic equivalents, especially when trying to conceive.

There is also a school of thought that believes organic food may be better nutritionally, but this is still being researched.

Foresight stresses the dangers of environmental toxins, identifying at least 200 man-made chemicals for which there is evidence of reproductive hazards. The association also stresses that eating organic foods will at least help to reduce the risks of some of these chemicals.

Surrey University undertook some research on Foresight's work and studied a group of 367 couples who enrolled on the Foresight program due to number of different problems. Of these 367, 217 had infertility issues. Within one to three years, 327 of the group had successfully conceived healthy children. The success rate among the infertile couples in the group was 86 per cent.

Eating organic food is just one of the recommendations made by Foresight; a considerable number of other factors also play a part in successful conception. *See* pages 38-39 for more information about organic foods.

staying healthy

Being underweight or overweight can have an affect on conception...

weight

Achieving and maintaining an ideal body weight is important both to general health and fertility. Being underweight or overweight can have an affect on conception—*see* pages 78-9, or consult a registered nutritionist, dietician, or your doctor for more information on ideal weights.

In addition, research has indicated that excessive dieting and overeating can contribute to infertility problems.

If women are overweight, they can stop ovulating. Studies have shown that losing even a little weight can be sufficient to increase fertility by stimulating ovulation, improving hormone balance, and making periods more regular.

Consequently, experts advise achieving an ideal body weight by eating a healthy and nutritious diet (*see* pages 34-61). Women should also aim to maintain that weight for as long as possible prior to conception. This allows their bodies the chance to achieve the balance of hormones that will maximize the chances of conceiving (*Ref 1.18*).

contraceptive pill

The pill interferes with the hormone system to prevent pregnancy. Bear in mind that it may take your body a little time to start producing these hormones again once you have stopped taking the pill (*Ref 1.19*). Foresight usually recommends mineral testing and readjustment after the use of this form of contraception (*Ref 1.20*).

fertility:
what to avoid

There is much evidence to suggest that toxic metals can be harmful to the body and have a negative effect on fertility levels.

toxic metals

Toxic metals are defined as "those elements not recognized as having an essential function and known to have well-documented deleterious effects" (Ref. 1.21).

There is much evidence to suggest that toxic metals can be harmful to the body and may have a negative effect on fertility levels. The key toxic metals on which research has been focused include the following.

lead

Lead, which comes, for example, from water that flows through lead pipes, was used in the past to induce an abortion (Ref. 1.22).

Men exposed to high levels of lead in the workplace have been found to be at risk of low sperm counts, with a greater number of sperm likely to be misshapen and less mobile (Ref. 1.23).

mercury

Mercury is found in pesticides, fungicides, fish, dental fillings, and industrial processes. Female dental assistants and female dentists exposed to mercury through the fillings they handle have been found to be less fertile than females who don't come into contact with the metal (*Ref. 1.24*).

For example. The UK Department of Health recommends that pregnant women do not have mercury fillings put in place during pregnancy.

cadmium

Cadmium is an inorganic poison present in tobacco smoke, processed foods, manufacturing industries, shellfish from polluted waters, and galvanized containers. It accumulates in the body, and blocks nutrients such as zinc, which is critical for both male and female fertility.

Cadmium blocks nutrients such as zinc, which is critical for both male and female fertility.

aluminum

Aluminum, found in indigestion tablets, cookware, or foil and in canned drinks, dried milk substitutes, and deodorants, can be absorbed by the skin.

copper

Copper can be both toxic and beneficial, depending on the amount of exposure to it. Your body absorbs copper from water pipes, contraceptive coils, swimming pools, and jewelry. Copper can become increased in concentration in the body after hormonal treatments, such as the contraceptive pill or fertility drugs.

assessing your toxins

In order to assess the levels of toxic metals present in the body, it is worth contacting a registered nutritionist or dietician to arrange a personal consultation so that tests can be organized and a plan of action structured to your own individual needs

A nutritionist will help identify the source of contamination, which will then need to be avoided if possible. In addition, they may recommend taking specific nutrients such as antioxidants (vitamin C, for example) to help eliminate toxins from the body.

The liver detoxifies the body by combining harmful substances (e.g., chemicals, drugs, alcohol, heavy toxic metals) with less harmful substances, which are then excreted by the kidneys. Making sure the liver is working as healthily and as efficiently as possible will help eliminate heavy toxins and other unwanted substances. Seek advice on ways of doing this.

caffeine

Caffeine is more widely used than many people expect. In addition to tea and coffee, caffeine is also present in chocolate, soft drinks, and medicines—particularly some widely available headache remedies.

Caffeine is a diuretic, causing its user to pass more urine than normal and potentially flushing away vital nutrients that are important to fertility.

Ideally, aim to eliminate caffeine altogether or reduce your intake of it to the lowest possible level. This may be achieved gradually to reduce the unpleasant effects of withdrawal such as headaches, tiredness, or depression.

Caffeine is a diuretic, causing its user to pass more urine than normal and potentially flushing away vital nutrients that are important to fertility.

food additives

Food additives come in the form of preservatives and artificial colorings, flavorings, and, sweeteners, to name but a few. There are over 4,000 additives—both artificial and natural—in use in the UK alone. To date, very little research has been carried out on the effects of additives before and during pregnancy. Consequently, organizations such as the Foresight association recommend avoiding additives prior to conception. It is certainly a good idea to avoid all artificial additives if at all possible. Choosing organic foods can go some way to helping achieve this.

alcohol

Most of us have heard that drinking and smoking while pregnant can be harmful to the baby. What most of us may not realize is that smoking and alcohol can reduce fertility.

Research has shown that drinking alcohol causes a decrease in sperm counts, and an increase in abnormal sperm (Ref. 1.25).

In addition, alcohol can prevent the absorption of nutrients such as zinc, which is regarded as one of the most important minerals for male virility.

Fetal alcohol syndrome (FAS) was originally defined by a group of medical researchers in the US. It has now been more clearly defined by international research, and the abnormalities of a baby suffering from FAS range from being underweight and under-length at birth to having slow growth and a failure to thrive after birth even with special postnatal care. Additional potential problems include possible mental retardation and/or behavioral problems such as hyperactivity and extreme nervousness.

For maximum safety and optimum development in the child, Foresight (see page 9) advises a complete embargo on alcohol for both parents in the four months leading up to the intended conception, and for the mother throughout pregnancy and breastfeeding.

The UK Department of Health advises that women trying to become pregnant should drink no more than one or two units—a unit is one glass of wine or half a pint of beer—of alcohol once or twice a week and should avoid heavy drinking sessions. The same advice comes from the UK's Health Development Agency.

In a study in Denmark, Dr. Tina Kold Jensen and colleagues from the National University Hospital studied 430 Danish couples aged 20 to 35 years who were trying to have a baby for the first time. The results of the study were published in the British Medical Journal.

In this study, women who consumed an average of 11 to 15 drinks a week during a cycle had only a third of the chance of conceiving that month as women who avoided alcohol altogether. Moderate drinkers—those who had six to 10 drinks a week—were half as likely to conceive. Even light drinkers—those who had one to five drinks a week—cut their chances of becoming pregnant by a third.

If you are trying to conceive, it makes sense to refrain from drinking or at least limit your intake (Ref 1.26).

tobacco

When smoked, tobacco produces more than 4,000 compounds including carbon monoxide, oxides of nitrogen, ammonia, aromatic hydrocarbons, hydrogen cyanide, vinyl chloride, lead, and cadmium, in addition to nicotine.

Cigarette smoking has been linked to infertility problems in both women (*Refs 1.28 & 1.29*) and men (*Ref 1.27*).

Smoking has also been linked to problems in pregnancy and childbirth. Premature babies are seen to be born more often to mothers who smoke compared to those who don't. Similarly, studies have found that smokers are more likely to give birth to children with all types of congenital malformations.

For example, the "Oxford Survey on Childhood Cancers", published in 1997 in the *British Journal of Cancer*, found that men who smoke when their partners don't still run a higher risk of fathering children who develop cancer. The survey stated that one in seven childhood cancers, including leukemia and brain tumors, could be due to the father's smoking habits.

It is advisable to stop smoking at least four months prior to conception, and to avoid smoky atmospheres as much as possible.

It is advisable to stop smoking at least four months prior to conception.

drugs

The use of street drugs such as cocaine and marijuana has increased steadily over the years. Many drugs have been associated with infertility and, if taken during pregnancy, may bring about problems with the unborn baby's health and development. Babies born to mothers who have taken certain drugs during pregnancy can also suffer withdrawal symptoms (often severe).

Research indicates that if women take such drugs during pregnancy, they risk giving birth to babies with low birth weights or malformations, as well as being more prone to miscarriages and stillbirths (Ref 1.30).

If you are addicted to a street drug, seek professional help by talking to your doctor, who can then refer you to a specialist to help overcome the problem. It is recommended that women eliminate all drugs from their bodies at least four months before conception.

The Foresight Association (see page 9) also recommends avoiding the use of all over-the-counter drugs such as laxatives, painkillers, etc., where possible, before and during pregnancy. The association believes that by paying attention to your diet you can help to eliminate the need for this sort of medication.

It does not matter what the drug is; it will always have an unnatural effect on the body's biochemistry (Ref 1.31).

It does not matter what the drug is; it will always have an unnatural effect on the body's biochemistry.

excessive exercise

Everyone should aim to incorporate some form of exercise into his or her lifestyle to help stay healthy and in shape. Before and during pregnancy, this advice is no different. You should adapt your exercise routine to suit your base level of fitness. Excessive exercise—any exercise that places extreme physical stress on the body and lowers body fat to below what is needed to maintain normal menstrual function—is not advisable, either before and during pregnancy.

Menstrual disorders have been reported in underweight athletic women and also in women with eating disorders such as anorexia nervosa.

Good forms of gentle exercise include walking, swimming and yoga.

pregnancy diet

pregnancy
care

eating during pregnancy

...many experts have been able to show a definite link between a newborn baby's health and its mother's diet during pregnancy.

During pregnancy, what you eat and drink will invariably affect the health and development of another little person.

Take the opportunity to have a thorough look at your diet and make any necessary changes to help reach your optimum health. If you are strong and healthy, there is a stronger chance that you will produce a strong and healthy baby. In the myriad studies on relationships between diet and pregnancy, many experts have been able to show a definite link between a newborn baby's health and its mother's diet during pregnancy.

During its time in the womb, a baby is completely dependent on its mother for the nutrients it needs to grow and develop. With most nutrients, the baby's needs tend to be met before the mother's. While this is good news for the developing baby, it is still important that expectant mothers achieve the recommended nutrient intakes from their diet to help prevent any problems with general health, such as brittle hair, bad teeth, sallow skin, etc.

Some mothers may experience challenges such as fatigue, morning sickness, cramps, anemia, etc., many of which can be greatly reduced or even avoided altogether with a good diet.

To help you work toward a healthy diet, take a look at the following recommended guidelines and see if you can work them into your diet. The rest of the chapter looks at a list of specific nutrients in detail.

• Enjoy your food. Don't give up any of the foods you enjoy most.
• Eat a variety of different foods. No one food contains all the nutrients needed in the right amounts, so eat a mixture of foods to get the right amount of a good range of nutrients.
• Choose foods from the following five food groups.
1 Bread, cereals, and potatoes. This includes breakfast cereals, granola, oats, pasta, noodles, sweet potatoes, and cornmeal.
2 Fruit and vegetables. This group includes salads and fresh and frozen fruits.
3 Milk and dairy. This includes yogurt, milk, and cheese
4 Meat, fish, and alternatives. This group covers fresh and frozen fish, lamb, pork, and beef, eggs, beans, lentils, and nuts.
5 Foods containing fat and sugar. Foods in this group include butter and oil, cakes, cookies, desserts, and other sweets.

Foods from the first four groups should be eaten every day, while foods in the fifth group are best not eaten too often or in large amounts. It is also important to choose a variety of foods from each group, rather than just eating the same type each time, in order to get a mixture of all the different nutrients.

• Eat plenty of foods rich in starch and fiber. These include bread, cereals, sweet potatoes, cornmeal, sweet corn, millet, noodles, pasta, and rice. They are the main sources of starch and fiber, but they also provide other nutrients as well. Many people believe that these foods are fattening, which is not true. It is how we cook or serve them that adds on the calories. For example, a slice of bread with a scraping of butter on the top has twice as many calories as a slice of bread on its own.
• Eat plenty of fresh fruits and vegetables. Try to eat five servings a day. This is not as difficult as it may first appear. The five servings include *both* fruits and vegetables, not five servings of each.

fruits & vegetables

When you think about a good, healthy day's diet, it becomes clear just how easy this is to achieve. For example, for breakfast, drink a fruit smoothie (whizz together a banana, handful of strawberries, and milk to taste) or have a selection of fresh fruits, chopped up and served on cereal. For lunch, enjoy a mixed crunchy salad with a yogurt dressing served with a baked potato. Make sure supper includes some vegetables, whether it is a quick stir-fry or a few steamed green vegetables to go with fish. Don't forget a few pieces of fruit to munch on during the day as quick snacks.

cut down on fats

Don't eat too many foods that contain a lot of fat. We all need a small amount of fat in our diets, as it is essential for health, but we need to eat more of the right sorts of fats—unsaturates—and less of the saturates such as butter, lard, and cakes. Use vegetable or nut oils for cooking and dressings and eat oily fish twice a week to provide the essential fats important for building an unborn baby's brain, eyes, and nerves (*see* pages 44 for more information about fats).

Don't have sugary foods and drinks too often. Too much sugar in the diet can contribute to an excess energy intake, which can lead to obesity. Avoid cakes, cookies, pastries, jams, marmalades, and syrups as much as possible. Instead, add sweetness to foods with ingredients such as dried and fresh fruits.

raw foods

Raw food—for example, fresh fruits, vegetables, nuts, and sprouted seeds—are great nutrient-dense foods. As cooking these foods destroys some of their nutritional value, it is a good idea to incorporate raw foods into your daily diet.

Another advantage of eating foods in their raw state is that they contain more water raw than when they are cooked. In contrast to water obtained from the faucet or from bottles, the water in raw foods contains much-needed nutrients such as vitamins, proteins, electrolytes, amino acids, carbohydrates, and fatty acids. Water also increases cell metabolism and helps boost energy levels. It is possible that food sensitivities and digestive disturbances may be reduced by eating raw foods.

Eating foods in such a natural state may calm the digestive system. It is no coincidence that diets rich in natural, nonprocessed, or unrefined foods have also been linked to longevity.

It is very easy to include raw foods in the diet by making small changes to the way you eat. For example, pack salad ingredients into sandwiches, sprinkle nuts and seeds over salads, and enjoy more fresh fruits by whizzing them together in a food processor to make a smoothie.

When it is not possible to use raw foods, use fast methods of cooking such as steaming and stir-frying.

It is possible that food sensitivities and digestive disturbances may be reduced by eating raw foods. Eating foods in such a natural state may calm the digestive system.

Phytochemicals have been shown to help protect against cancer and heart disease. Since the body cannot store them, it is a good idea to eat as many fresh fruits and vegetables as possible.

phytochemicals

Research continues to provide reasons for eating more raw fruit and vegetables. The most recently discovered natural plant substances are known as "phytochemicals," "phyto" meaning "plant" in Greek. Phytochemicals are compounds found in food that interact in complex, complementary ways.

Phytochemicals are given weird and wonderful names that you may well come across on ingredient labels and in health magazines. Of the known health-enhancing phytochemicals, better-known examples include bioflavonoids, plant sterols, chlorophyll, and phenols.

These substances can have a major impact on your life. Certain phytochemicals have been shown to help protect against cancer and heart disease. Since the body cannot store phytochemicals, it is a good idea to eat as many fresh fruits and vegetables as possible—aiming for the recommended five portions (combined) of fresh fruits and vegetables a day to reap the full benefits that these substances provide.

Recent research comparing the effectiveness of taking supplements versus naturally occurring foods indicates that the body is able to make better use of naturally occurring foods. This is quite possibly due to the complex set of chemical reactions that occur among all the enzymes, vitamins, minerals, amino acids, and phytochemicals. Put simply, raw, organic food is the most natural and beneficial way of getting nutrients and vitamins into the body.

organic foods

"Organic" refers not to the food itself, but to how it is produced. Organic is a legal term, and all organic food production and processing is governed by strict guidelines.

The aim of organic farming and the philosophy behind it is to be a safe, sustainable system of farming that produces healthy crops and livestock without damaging the environment.

Eating organic foods can help limit your intake of toxins such as pesticide residues and additives that could be passed on to your unborn baby. The negative cumulative effects of these substances on humans are not yet known. However, many experts believe that babies are more at risk from these toxins than adults, especially during the first few weeks of life inside the womb, when their tiny vital organs and limbs are still developing.

Some advantages of eating organic foods before and during pregnancy include the following.

● They are free from genetically modified organisms.
● Nearly all organic foods are free from pesticide residues.
● They do not contain artificial additives such as chemical sweeteners or emulsifiers and "E-numbers"; however, be aware that they may contain natural added ingredients such as sugars, salts, thickening agents, etc.
● Organic meat is free from growth promoters or hormones and contains very few, if any, antibiotics. In non-organic dairy foods, by comparison, excessive levels of antibiotics have been found. It is thought that these may cause the development of resistant strains of bacteria in babies and young children.
● Organic meat has never been reported as having a single case of BSE (mad cow disease).
● Some evidence suggests that organic foods may be richer in nutrients than their non-organic equivalents, although this is still being researched. Organic farmers use traditional methods of farming such as crop rotation and green manure to ensure that the soil is given the chance to replace

Eating organic foods can help limit your intake of toxins such as pesticide residues and additives that could be passed on to your unborn baby.

nutrients taken by the previous crops, so the argument does seem valid. Also, organic fruit and vegetables are not waxed to prolong shelf life; hence their skins—often a good source of nutrients—are safe to eat.

• The flavor of organic foods tends to be better than their non-organic equivalents. This is due partly to the fact that organic foods tend to be picked when fully ripe. Also, unlike conventionally grown fruits and vegetables, they are not fed with artificial fertilizers, which encourage the plants to take up more water, resulting in a more "diluted" taste.

In the UK, farms wishing to market organic products are inspected by various bodies which have been approved by the UK Register of Organic Food Standards to check that high standards are being maintained. Producers and farmers are subject to rigid testing, including soil testing, before certification is granted; 70 to 80 per cent of approved producers are certified by the Soil Association. It takes a minimum of two years for a farm to gain organic status. During this time, the farm needs to develop the soil's natural fertility and allow pesticide residues to diminish.

For these and many other reasons, aim to include as much organic food as possible in your diet.

The flavor of organic foods tends to be better than their non-organic equivalents. This is due partly to the fact that organic foods tend to be picked when fully ripe.

pregnancy nutrition

If individuals consume the RNI of a nutrient, they are very unlikely to be deficient in that nutrient.

This section includes information about the different nutrients found in your diet. As a guide, 50 per cent of your daily calorie intake should come from carbohydrates; 33 to 35 per cent from all fats, including a maximum 10 per cent of saturated fats; and 12 per cent from protein.

The recommended quantities of all nutrients for pregnant women are given by the UK's Department of Health (DOH) as reference nutrient intakes, or "RNIs".

recommended nutrient intake (RNI)

Defined by the UK's DOH as an amount of a nutrient that is enough for over 97 per cent of people, even those with high needs for the nutrient. Consequently, the RNI is a higher amount of a nutrient than most people need. According to the DOH, "If individuals consume the RNI of a nutrient, they are very unlikely to be deficient in that nutrient."

nutritional units of measurement

g	gram	
mg	milligram	one thousandth of 1 g
mcg	microgram	one-millionth of 1 g
ng	nanogram	one-billion of 1 g
kg	kilogram	1,000 g
kcal	kilocalorie	1 calorie (unit used to measure the energy value of food)

energy

The amount of energy you have is partly dependent on the foods you eat. Your diet needs to feature plenty of good fats, carbohydrates, and protein—the building blocks of energy. However, you need to limit your intake of processed foods, which may contain relatively high amounts of bad fats and sugars but very little else.

Energy is measured in calories (cals) or kilocalories (kcals).

why you need energy during pregnancy

Energy is required to both support the growth of the fetus and to enable fat to be deposited in women's bodies for use when they are breastfeeding.

how much you need

Individual calorie requirements vary enormously. Energy requirements are determined largely by the amount of energy you use, your basal metabolic rate (the rate at which your body uses energy while at complete rest), and any special needs, for example, pregnancy and breastfeeding.

Energy needed to maintain your basal metabolic rate includes energy to maintain body temperature and other normal functions such as heartbeat and breathing. If your energy intake from food is greater than your total energy use, the balance will be turned into fat and stored as an energy reserve.

Energy is needed during pregnancy to support the growing fetus and to enable fat to be deposited in the mother's body, ready for lactation. However reductions occur in physical activity and metabolic rate which help compensate for increased needs.

Consequently, the need to increase energy intakes during pregnancy is limited to a small amount during the last trimester only. The increase in estimated average requirement* (EAR) above pre-pregnancy intake is 200 kcal a day for the final three months only (weeks 27 to 40). However, women who are underweight at the beginning of pregnancy may need to eat more.

where you get it

Good sources of energy include vegetables, fruit, cereals, meat, fish, and dairy products, which supply energy as well as essential nutrients. Poor sources include highly processed foods such as cakes, pastries, and chocolate, which can contain high amounts of hidden sugar and fat and often few or no essential nutrients. These provide "empty" calories. Having sufficient calories is important, but these calories need to come from the good sources.

* Estimated Average Requirement

The Estimated Average Requirement for energy

15- to 18-year-old females	2,110 kcal/day
19- to 49-year-old females	1,940 kcal/day
50- to 59-year-old females	1,900 kcal/day

There are two types of carbohydrates: simple (sugars) and complex (starches and fibers). They are the body's primary source of energy. Carbohydrates should account for two-thirds of the calories you consume.

Simple carbohydrates, found in foods such as candy and chocolate, are high in calories and provide instant energy. When you eat sugar, your blood-sugar level rises, causing your body to release insulin into the bloodstream to stabilize this raised level. It is important to keep blood-sugar levels balanced in order to maintain energy levels.

When blood sugar is low, you may feel hungry, tired, depressed, or lack concentration. When it is high—after a sugary snack—the release of insulin triggers a rapid drop in blood sugar, which makes you feel tired and hungry again. When there are high levels of sugar in the blood, the body converts the excess (in the short term) to glycogen, or to fat for long-term energy storage.

It is important to keep blood-sugar levels balanced in order to maintain energy levels.

carbohydrates

source	carbohydrates/100g	starch/100g	sugar/100g
Whole-wheat bread	41.6 g	39.8 g	1.8 g
Potatoes	17.2 g	16.6 g	0.6 g
Brown rice	81.3 g	80.0 g	1.3 g
White rice	85.8 g	85.8 g	trace
Bananas	23.2 g	2.3 g	20.9 g
Chickpeas, canned	16.1 g	15.1 g	0.4 g
Puffed wheat	67.3 g	67.0 g	0.3 g

High levels of insulin inhibit the breakdown of fat. Diabetes develops when the body cannot produce enough insulin to regulate blood sugar. This leads to a high blood-sugar level and not enough glucose going to other organs in the body.

Complex carbohydrates (starches and fibers) are found in foods such as whole grains, rice, potatoes, and vegetables. Our bodies have to work hard to digest starches—even harder if they are unrefined, such as whole-wheat bread, pasta, and brown rice. This slows down our metabolisms, provides long-lasting energy, and helps to keep blood-sugar levels constant.

The energy in food is measured in calories. Carbohydrates provide nearly four calories per gram.

Most of your extra calories during the last three months of pregnancy should come from carbohydrates.

why you need carbohydrate during pregnancy

Carbohydrates help to provide the fetus with the supply of energy it needs for growth. Most of the extra calories needed during the last three months of pregnancy should come from carbohydrates.

how much you need

The requirement for carbohydrates is not affected by pregnancy. However, to maintain good health, you should eat more unrefined or "complex" carbohydrates, which means more starchy and high-fiber foods. You should also consume less sugar and fewer high-sugar foods.

where to get it

Good sources of carbohydrates include whole grains, rice, bread, fruits, and vegetables. Poor sources of carbohydrates include processed foods such as cookies, pastries, and chocolate.

fat

Essential fatty acids are vital for the brain and nervous system, cardiovascular system, and skin.

Fats and oils are made up of molecules of fatty acids and glycerol. All fats are made up of a combination of three types of fatty acid. A fat is said to be saturated, monounsaturated, or poly-unsaturated, depending on which type of fatty acid is present in largest proportion. Saturated fats such as butter, are solid at room temperature. Monounsaturated fats, like olive oil, are liquid at room temperature. Polyunsaturated fats, such as sunflower oil, are liquid at room temperature and they also remain liquid even when it is cold.

Some fatty acids in the diet are absolutely essential to health. These essential fatty acids, or EFAs, are found in plant and fish oils. They are known as linoleic acid and linolenic acid. Such essential fatty acids cannot be made in the body, so, like vitamins and minerals, they need to be eaten in the diet.

Fats are much higher in calories than either protein or carbohydrate. There are nine kilocalories (kcal) in every gram of fat, compared to four per gram of protein, or 3.75 per gram of carbohydrates.

why you need fat during pregnancy

Some fat is essential in everyone's diet. Foods that contain fats provide a concentrated source of energy, and the fat-soluble vitamins A, D, E, and K. These vitamins are vital for normal growth and development.

Essential fatty acids are vital for the brain and nervous system, immune system, cardiovascular system, and skin; hence, they are necessary during pregnancy to help ensure the proper development of the baby.

Essential fats have also been found to be crucial for development of the baby's brain, eyes, and central nervous system (*Ref. 2.1*). A good supply can help to prevent low birth weights and decrease the likelihood of a premature birth with all its potential risks, including cerebral palsy, blindness, deafness, etc. (*Ref. 2.2*).

how much you need

Unlike most other nutrients, there is no requirement, as such, for fats. However, the British Nutrition Foundation Task Force and the World Health Organization have recommended that women planning pregnancy, and those already pregnant, should have an adequate intake of essential fatty acids. Most authorities now agree that fat should constitute about 35 per cent of the energy content of your diet, with no more than 10 per cent coming from animal sources.

An optimum amount of essential fatty acids required for pregnancy is not known. But it is thought that, on the whole, most people living in developed countries already get sufficient to satisfy their needs. However, recent surveys have shown that many people's diets are low in linoleic acid, one of the important essential fats (see right).

where to get it

Saturated fats come mainly from animal products such as butter, lard, suet, dripping, meat, eggs, whole milk, cheese, and yoghurt made from whole milk. Saturated fats are also found in hard margarines (hydrogenated vegetable oil), which contain trans-fatty acids (see below). Also high in saturated fats are coconut oil and palm oil.

Unsaturated fats are generally liquid at room temperature and come from vegetable sources, particularly oils, e.g. olive, sunflower, soy, peanut, and sesame. Linolenic acid and linoleic acid are also found in oils, e.g sesame, safflower, soy, and corn oil, as well as in nuts, seeds, fatty fish (herring, mackerel, sardines, and salmon), and soy drinks.

Margarines and low-fat spreads often contain hydrogenated vegetable oil. Hydrogenation involves transforming the vegetable oil into a solid fat by changing its chemical structure (it becomes a trans-fatty acid). It was once thought that all vegetable fats, solid or liquid, had fewer detrimental health effects than animal fats. However, research indicates that trans-fatty acids can cause free-radical damage—linked with heart disease and cancer— within the body's cells. Now some soft margarines have the trans-fatty acids removed.

In preference to hard margarine, use olive oil or a small amount of butter.

During pregnancy, protein is required not only for the growth of the baby, but also for the growth of other protein-rich tissues.

Protein consists of building blocks called amino acids. There are two types of amino acids: essential and nonessential. Essential amino acids must be obtained directly from food, while the body can produce non-essential amino acids from other sources. You therefore need to make sure that your diet contains enough essential amino acids.

why you need protein during pregnancy

Protein is needed to help the body build or repair muscles, tissues, hair, and organs, and to maintain an effective immune and hormonal system. During pregnancy, protein is required not only for the growth of the baby, but also for the growth of other protein-rich tissues, including extra blood cells, the uterus in particular, and the placenta.

Proteins in the diet are broken down by digestive enzymes and absorbed into the blood as amino acids. These are then taken to build and repair cells and carry out their other roles, as required. Any extra protein may be used for energy or stored as fat. During pregnancy, protein is used efficiently: less protein is used for energy and more is stored for use by the baby.

protein

protein source	protein intake/source
2½ cups skim milk	19.80 g
6-oz salmon fillet, steamed	35.18 g
8-oz sirloin steak (lean and fat), raw	37.35 g
1 cup tofu (soybean curd), steamed	18.23 g
1¾ oz Cheddar cheese	12.75 g
1⅛ cups green or brown lentils, boiled in salted water	22.00 g
1½ cups white rice, boiled	6.00 g

how much you need

Some experts recommend 54 g of protein a day. This increases by 11 per cent for pregnant women, or six grams per day. However, some nutritionists consider this estimate to be too high. The overall need for protein depends on both the quality of the protein, and the dietary intake of vitamins and minerals. This determines how efficiently you use protein. In other words, if you eat good-quality protein and are not vitamin and mineral deficient, you can afford to eat less than this. The minimum requirement for protein during pregnancy is 49 g per day.

where to get it

The best-quality protein foods (in terms of their amino-acid balance) include eggs, soybeans, meat, fish, dairy products, and poultry. Vegetarian protein foods, such as legumes, whole grains, nuts, seeds, and manufactured vegetable protein foods, don't contain all the essential amino acids, but if eaten in combination—legumes with grains, legumes with nuts, or nuts with seeds—they can meet the body's daily protein needs.

For example, good protein-providing vegetarian meals include lentil soup with whole-wheat bread, vegetable kebabs with nut sauces, and vegetable and cheese omelettes.

Unborn babies cannot make protein, so if mothers do not eat enough, they have to go without.

The following excellent-quality protein foods all provide about 20 g of protein: 4 cups brown rice, ⅔ cup canned tuna, ⅔ cup sardines, two medium eggs, 1¾ cups of yogurt, and 1 cup tofu (soybean curd).

Unborn babies cannot make protein, so if mothers do not eat enough, they have to go without.

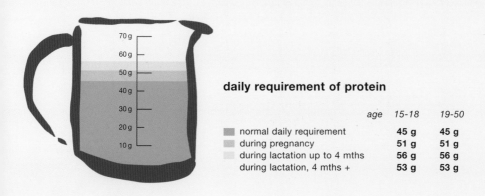

daily requirement of protein

	age	15-18	19-50
normal daily requirement		45 g	45 g
during pregnancy		51 g	51 g
during lactation up to 4 mths		56 g	56 g
during lactation, 4 mths +		53 g	53 g

Minerals are essential for almost every bodily process. For example, oxygen is carried in the blood by an iron compound; a lack of this mineral can lead to anemia. Calcium, magnesium, and phosphorus help make up bones and teeth.

Magnesium, calcium, and zinc, are important both before and during pregnancy. Research has shown that there is no increased need for other minerals during pregnancy. In developed countries, normal intakes are generally well above the recommended intake, so there is very little likelihood of anyone in the population being deficient in them. Such minerals include sodium chloride, potassium, copper, iodine, selenium, manganese, fluoride, chromium, nickel, and silicon.

Ninety-nine per cent of the body's calcium content is found in bones and teeth, with one per cent in blood plasma and soft tissues. The major part of phosphorus in the body is associated with calcium in the bones.

> Calcium, magnesium, and phosphorus help make up bones and teeth.

why you need calcium during pregnancy

Calcium is crucial for the formation of both healthy teeth and bones in an unborn baby.

calcium & phosphorus

calcium source	calcium intake/source
2½ cups skim milk	680 mg
2 tbsp almonds	96 mg
1¾ oz Cheddar cheese	360 mg
1½ oz (3) dried figs	112.5 mg
1 tbsp sesame seeds	134 mg
½ cup strained plain yogurt	200 mg
⅓ cup sardines canned in oil	275 mg

phosphorus source	phosphorus intake/source
2½ cups skim milk	540 mg
2 tbsp almonds	220 mg
1¾ oz Cheddar cheese	245 mg
1½ oz (3) dried figs	40 mg
1 tbsp sesame seeds	144 mg
½ cup strained plain yogurt	170 mg
⅓ cup sardines canned in oil	260 mg

how much calcium you need

The US FDA recommends 800 mg for adults and 1,200 mg for pregnant women and young adults.

During pregnancy, calcium absorption increases, but no additional calcium is generally needed. One exception is the pregnant adolescent, whose bone mineralization (hardening) may still be taking place. Consequently, the needs for dietary calcium both for herself and for the developing baby are particularly high.

Calcium concentrations are higher in a developing fetus than in its mother, which suggests that the baby will maintain an adequate supply at the mother's expense.

how much phosphorus you need

The US FDA recommends 800 mg for adults over 25 years of age and 1,200 mg for young adults and pregnant women.

where to get calcium & phosphorus

Both are found in the following foods. Almost half our calcium is obtained from milk and cheese, and a quarter comes from bread and other cereals. Just 2½ cups of milk daily will provide a just under the recommended intake. Other good sources include yogurt, tofu, and soy drinks enriched with calcium, canned fish (where the bones are eaten, such as sardines) and salmon, dark-green, leafy vegetables, dried fruit, nuts, and seeds, especially sesame seeds.

It is vital to include other trace minerals and vitamins, such as vitamin D, in the diet to make sure that calcium is absorbed and used by the body. Alcohol and caffeine can inhibit its absorption.

Vegans should pay particular attention to their calcium intakes to ensure adequate levels.

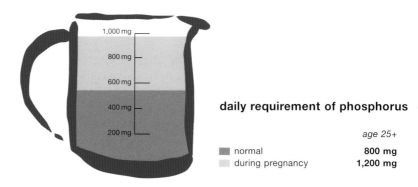

1,000 mg	
800 mg	
600 mg	
400 mg	
200 mg	

daily requirement of phosphorus

age 25+

▮ normal	**800 mg**
▮ during pregnancy	**1,200 mg**

zinc

Helping to maintain a healthy immune system and assisting in cell replication are just some of the functions of zinc.

Vitamins A, E, and B_6 as well as magnesium, calcium, and phosphorus all help the body to absorb zinc. Stress, alcohol, and a low-protein intake can prevent it from being absorbed. If we become deficient in zinc, we may experience acne or greasy skin, loss of appetite, and maybe depression.

why you need zinc during pregnancy

Zinc is involved in the process of cell replication. It is therefore important to have a good supply in the early stages of pregnancy.

A number of studies have found that women with low zinc levels had a greater tendency to have babies with congenital malformations of the central nervous system (Ref. 2.3). Low intakes early in pregnancy have been related to growth retardation and lower birth weights (Ref 2.4). See "Zinc" pages 16–7.

how much you need

Extra zinc is required during pregnancy, but women absorb this mineral more efficiently during pregnancy. The American diet is slightly low in zinc so the FDA recommendation for zinc intake is 30 mg of zinc daily in pregnancy and 15 mg for all other adults.

Long-term use of contraceptive pills may inhibit the absorption of zinc and cause the body to excrete more. Evidence of this is slight, but it is still recommended that women should make a real effort to eat a healthy diet with foods that contain zinc if they have just come off the pill.

where to get it

Sources include red meat, shellfish—mussels, crab, and lobster—canned sardines, turkey, Parmesan cheese, and other hard or crumbly cheeses (such as cheddar), nuts and seeds (including peanut butter and tahini), whole-grain cereals, legumes (dried peas, beans, and lentils), green vegetables such as watercress and spinach, and dried apricots, figs, and raisins.

zinc source	zinc intake/source
7 oz roast beef	13.60 mg
5 anchovies, canned	0.64 mg
10 oz stewing lamb	19.70 mg
1 tbsp pine nuts	1.30 mg
½ cup green lentils	1.95 mg
7 oz crab meat (½ crab)	11.00 mg
8 oz stewing steak	19.60 mg

iron

Iron is needed for healthy blood and muscles, and is vital for cell respiration—the process by which cells generate energy. Lack of iron in the body leads to a common form of anemia.

why you need iron during pregnancy

About 40 per cent of women aged 18 to 34 have low blood iron stores. Menstrual losses account for the fact that a woman's iron needs are much greater than the iron needs of a man.

During pregnancy, the placenta can deliver large quantities of iron to the baby, even if doing so means depriving its mother of iron. If women are suffering from iron deficiency, it is often a result of poor nutrition.

how much you need

The FDA recommendation for adults is 10 mg a day, 15 mg for premenopausal women, and 30 mg for pregnant women. There are many women who are not reaching the target. Therefore it is important to try to achieve the recommended iron intake before becoming pregnant, to help prevent a deficiency during the pregnancy.

Requirements for iron are not increased during pregnancy. This is partly because there is no loss of iron through menstruation, and also because iron is absorbed more efficiently during pregnancy.

where to get it

The two sources of iron in the diet are heme iron from animal protein and nonheme iron from plant sources. The body finds it easier to absorb heme iron. We are capable of absorbing 20 to 40 per cent of the iron from meat and only five to 20 per cent available from vegetable sources. Consequently, women need to eat a lot more of the nonheme sources to obtain a good supply of iron.

Good sources of heme iron include meat; moderate sources include lean meat, chicken, and fish; and small amounts are found in milk.

Good sources of nonheme iron include cereals fortified with iron, whole-grain bread, dark-green, leafy vegetables (such as watercress, spinach, broccoli, and Savoy cabbage), nuts, legumes, seeds, figs, apricots, prunes, raisins, licorice, and dark chocolate. Vitamin C and folic acid aid in the absorption of iron, so it is advisable to eat good sources of these nutrients at the same time. Try to include good sources of these vitamins in the same meal as your iron source.

iron source	iron intake/source
3⅔ cup spinach, raw	2.31 mg
1 tbsp sesame seeds	2.08 mg
1 tbsp tahini paste	2.12 mg
1½ oz (3) dried figs	1.89 mg
8-oz rump steak, broiled	7.90 mg
2 cups Special K®	7.98 mg
1 tbsp oat or wheat bran	9.0 mg

magnesium

Magnesium is vital for the release of energy, building strong bones, teeth, and muscles, and regulating body temperature. It also helps the body absorb and metabolize other nutrients such as calcium and vitamin C.

why you need magnesium during pregnancy

Magnesium was the mineral most closely associated with birth weight in one study, which found that premature birth and the risk of low birth weight was increased with low intakes early in pregnancy (*Ref. 2.5*).

how much you need

The FDA recommends 280 mg for women, 350 mg for men, and 320 mg for pregnant women. The average female intake is 237 mg, so some women need to increase their dietary intake prior to conception.

The good news is that absorption of magnesium increases during pregnancy. In contrast, when women are breastfeeding, they need an extra 50 mg a day.

where to get it

Excellent sources of magnesium include whole-grain cereal products such as. whole-wheat bread, whole-wheat pasta,and brown rice; nuts, such as almonds and cashews; seeds; legumes; green, leafy vegetables, such as spinach; peas; sweetcorn; zucchini; parsnips; milk; yogurt; lean meat; dried figs; apricots; raisins; and bananas.

magnesium source	magnesium intake/source
1 oz (2 slices) whole-wheat bread	60.8 mg
½ cup brown rice	60.5 mg
1 tbsp sunflower seeds	78.0 mg
2 tbsp Brazil nuts	164.0 mg
¾ oz (4 pieces) rye crispbread	20.0 mg
1½ oz (3) dried figs	36.0 mg
1 tbsp wheat bran	104.0 mg

vitamins

Vitamins "turn-on" enzymes, which help to make all body processes happen. We need vitamins for a variety of functions. These include producing energy, balancing hormones, boosting the immune system, and making healthy skin. There are 13 essential vitamins in total, each with a special role to play. These can be divided into two groups: fat-soluble (A, D, E, and K) and water-soluble (C and B-complex). Water-soluble vitamins cannot be stored by the body, so foods containing these should be eaten daily. They can also be destroyed by overcooking, especially boiling vegetables or fruit in lots of water. It is best to eat fresh fruit and vegetables raw or lightly cooked.

Both B and C vitamins are necessary for turning food into energy. In addition, vitamins A, C, and E are all antioxidants, which help protect against cancer, heart disease, and pollution. Vitamin D also helps to control the body's calcium intake.

B VITAMINS

B-complex vitamins cover a large group of substances, including B_1 (thiamin), B_2 (riboflavin), B_3 (niacin), folic acid, B_5 (pantothenic acid), B_6 (pyridoxine), and B_{12} (cyanocobalamine). These vitamins play many roles including metabolizing food and converting it into energy, assisting in the production of red blood cells, and aiding the development and maintenance of a healthy nervous system.

B_1 thiamin

This vitamin helps the body to convert both protein and carbohydrate into energy. Vitamin B_1 is also used in brain function, and metabolism. Tiredness, weakness, and mood swings are classic symptoms of a vitamin B_1 deficiency.

why you need vitamin B_1 during pregnancy

Low intakes, of thiamin and vitamin B_3 (niacin), have been associated with lower birth weights.

In one study, mothers who had a low intake of thiamine and niacin had a nine-fold higher probability of having a low birth-weight baby compared to the mothers who had high intakes. The same picture emerged with several other B vitamins, including riboflavin and vitamin B_6 (Ref. 2.6).

how much you need

The FDA recommends 1.1 mg a day for women. However, they state that pregnant women who burn great amounts of energy may need more than the adult RDA of thiamine.

Other B vitamins assist in the absorption of thiamine. Tea, coffee, alcohol, cooking, and refined foods can all restrict thiamine absorption.

where to get it

Good sources include whole-grain or enriched breads; breakfast cereals; legumes (peas, beans, and lentils); brewer's yeast; peanut butter; wheat germ, green vegetables such as cabbage, Brussels sprouts, asparagus, and watercress; peppers; and tomatoes.

vitamin B_1 source	vitamin B_1 intake/source
1 tbsp + 1 tsp tahini paste	0.19 mg
1 tbsp sesame seeds	0.19 mg
1 tbsp sunflower seeds	0.32 mg
⅓ cup peanuts	0.57 mg
1½ cups baked potato	0.74 mg
7-oz pork loin	1.76 mg

B$_2$ riboflavin

Vitamin B$_2$, or riboflavin, plays an essential role in the release of energy from proteins, fats, and carbohydrates.

why you need riboflavin during pregnancy

Riboflavin requirements relate to protein requirements. An increase in protein requirements during pregnancy means an increased need for riboflavin.

how much you need

The FDA recommends 1.3 mg a day for women increasing to 1.6 mg during pregnancy. Research indicates that the intakes of some women, particularly those who are trying to lose weight, tend to be lower than the RDA. Make sure you are eating good sources of riboflavin both before and during pregnancy.

where to get it

Excellent sources include milk and milk products. Two and a half cups of milk provides all the riboflavin you need in a day. Other good sources include cereal products, wheat germ, meat and meat products, yogurt, cheese, eggs, sardines, soy products, brewer's yeast and yeast extracts, and green, leafy vegetables.

B$_3$ niacin

Vitamin B$_3$, or niacin works with thiamin and riboflavin in releasing energy from food.

why you need niacin during pregnancy

Niacin is essential for cell division, normal growth, healthy skin, brain and nerve function, the tongue, and digestive organs.

how much you need

The FDA recommends 17 mg a day for pregnant women. Like thiamin and riboflavin, niacin requirements are related to energy intake.

where to get it

Good sources include meat and meat products, whole-grain cereals and bread, oily fish, poultry, eggs, cheese, brewer's yeast and yeast extracts, legumes (peas, beans, and lentils), dried fruit, and nuts.

vitamin B$_2$ source	vitamin B$_2$ intake/source
2 tbsp almonds	0.30 mg
3½ oz (4) passion fruit	12.00 mg
1¼ oz (handful) mushrooms	0.25 mg
⅓ cup sardines	0.18 mg
7 oz duck, roasted	0.94 mg
1¾ oz Cheddar cheese	0.20 mg

vitamin B$_3$ source	vitamin B$_3$ intake/source
⅓ cup peanuts	6.90 mg
1¼ oz (handful) mushrooms	2.56 mg
⅓ cup smoked salmon	4.4 mg
½ cup tuna in brine	9.36 mg
3¾ oz chicken meat	11.30 mg
2 cups Special K®	12.00 mg
1 tbsp wheat bran	5.92 mg

B$_6$ pyridoxine

B$_{12}$ cobalamin

Vitamin B$_6$ is needed for growth, to convert protein into energy, protect against heart disease, regulate the menstrual cycle, and help with the functioning of the nervous and immune systems. B$_6$ supplementation can also help relieve premenstrual tension.

why you need vitamin B$_6$ during pregnancy

Vitamin B$_6$ and folic acid are frequently associated with pregnancy complications and adverse outcomes (Ref. 2.7). Vitamin B$_6$ is essential for breaking down protein for use in the growth of new body tissues and the production of antibodies and red blood cells.

how much you need

The RDA of vitamin B$_6$ for pregnant women is 2.2 mg and non-pregnant women is 1.6 mg per day. The average intake of vitamin B$_6$ from food is 1.6 mg per day. There are women whose intakes are below the recommended amount (Ref. 2.8).

where to get it

Good sources include meat, chicken, and fish. Others include whole-grain and enriched breads, breakfast cereals, brewer's yeast, potatoes, beans, lentils, green vegetables, bananas, melons, and peanuts.

Vitamin B$_{12}$ is linked with folic acid in having a central role in the production of red blood cells and the prevention of anemia.

why you need vitamin B$_{12}$ during pregnancy

Vitamin B$_{12}$ assists in maintaining the metabolism and the nervous system. It also aids in the prevention of pernicious anemia, and assists the proper formation of blood cells.

how much you need

The FDA recommends a daily intake of 2 mcg for adults and 2.2 mcg for pregnant women. Nursing women should also keep intakes up.

where to get it

It is found almost exclusively in foods of animal origin, e.g sardines, milk, cheese, and eggs. Vegans sources include fortified soy drinks or Marmite®.

vitamin B$_{12}$ source	vitamin B$_{12}$ intake/source
⅓ cup sardines, canned in oil	14.00 ug
7 oz duck, roasted	6.00 ug
½ cup tuna in brine	2.80 ug
2½ oz cod, baked	3.40 ug
8-oz beef steak	4.50 ug
2 medium-sized eggs, scrambled	2.52 ug

vitamin B$_6$ source	vitamin B$_6$ intake/source
1 tbsp sesame seeds	0.15 mg
2 tbsp hazelnuts	0.24 mg
5¼-oz (1 medium) banana	0.44 mg
7-oz (1 medium) avocado	0.72 mg
1½ cups baked potato	1.08 mg
14 oz chicken breast	2.12 mg
2 cups Special K®	1.32 mg

Folic acid plays a vital role in cell division and in creating healthy blood cells. It is also needed to enable the body to absorb iron—a nutrient needed for healthy blood.

why you need folic acid during pregnancy

Folic acid is important for the unborn baby's developing spinal cord. It is needed to make new cells and genetic material and, most importantly, aids in the prevention of neural tube defects (NTDs) such as spina bifida.

Spina bifida—a condition in which the spinal cord does not develop properly—has been strongly linked to a lack of folic acid. Folic acid is also needed to help prevent the development of certain types of anemia and promote the growth of fetal tissues and organs. It is also needed for the formation of protein tissues in the mother and the fetus.

how much you need

folic acid

Folic acid is important for the developing spinal cord. It helps make new cells and genetic material, and aids in the prevention of neural tube defects...

folic acid source	folic acid intake/source
⅓ cup peanuts	55.0 ug
1 tbsp sesame seeds	19.4 ug
6-oz (whole) orange	55.8 ug
3⅔ cups spinach, raw	165.0 ug
7 medium-sized spears of asparagus, boiled	155.0 ug
½ cup Brussels sprouts	93.5 ug
1½ cups baked potato	88.0 ug
2 cups Special K®	198.0 ug
½ cup brown rice	27.0 ug

The FDA recommends 180 mcg of folic acid a day for adult women. They recommend that all women of childbearing age, especially if planning to become pregnant or who may become pregnant should consume 400 mcg folic acid daily. (*Ref. 2.9*). The first 12 weeks are the most critical, because after this period the baby's neural tube will have passed through its most vulnerable period.

The average intake is between 109 and 203 ug per day, so eating foods rich in folic acid, as well as supplementation is essential to reach the total of 400 mcg.

A survey of 23,000 women showed that those who supplemented their diet with folic acid during the first six weeks of pregnancy had a 75 per cent lower incidence of NTDs than those who didn't (*Ref. 2.10*).

Genetics also play a part in NTDs—not all can be prevented by folic acid supplementation. If either parent has spina bifida, their risk of having a NTD baby is increased tenfold (*Ref. 2.11*). If there is a known case of a NTD, most commonly spina bifida, in either family, it is important to discuss this with your doctor before pregnancy.

where to get it

Folic acid occurs naturally in many foods, particularly plant foliage. Good sources include green, leafy vegetables—Savoy cabbage, Brussels sprouts, and spinach—broccoli, asparagus, whole-wheat bread, and cereal, dark yellow vegetables and fruit—oranges, grapefruit, mangoes, papaya, peaches, and pumpkin—beans, enriched grain products, and nuts. Try to eat much of your fresh vegetables and fruits raw, steamed, microwaved, or quickly stir-fried. Folic acid is destroyed by heat and leaks out into cooking water.

It is quite a challenge to achieve 400 mcg of folic acid through diet alone, so it is advisable to take a recommended supplement.

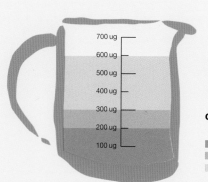

700 ug
600 ug
500 ug
400 ug
300 ug
200 ug
100 ug

daily requirement of folic acid

normal daily requirement	180 mcg
during pregnancy	400 mcg
whilst planning pregnancy	400 mcg

One of the antioxidant vitamins, Vitamin C is needed for a variety of functions: helping to turn food into energy; strengthening the immune system; keeping bones and joints strong; growth and healthy body tissue; healing wounds; and the absorption of iron (see page 51). Deficiency in vitamin C can result in a lack of energy, colds, bleeding or tender gums, and slow healing of wounds.

vitamin C source	vitamin C intake/source
⅔ cup strawberries	77.0 mg
6-oz (whole) orange	97.2 mg
½ cup kiwi fruit	50.2 mg
½ cup guava	172.5 mg
1 cup black currants	200.0 mg
4 cups turnip greens, raw	120.0 mg
7-oz (whole medium) red bell pepper	280.0 mg

vitamin c

why you need vitamin C during pregnancy

Vitamin C assists the absorption of iron from plant sources. A deficiency can have a negative effect on the production of collagen—a protein needed for bone structure, cartilage, muscle, and blood vessels.

Vitamin C levels in fetal blood may be 50 per cent higher than in the mother's blood. The placenta has the ability to concentrate some nutrients to the benefit of the fetus.

how much you need

The FDA recommends 60 mg a day for adult women, increasing to 70 mg per day for pregnant women and 70 mg per day during breastfeeding. A slight vitamin C deficiency is fairly common in the US today but severe deficiencies are rare.

Remember that vitamin C is a water-soluble vitamin which cannot be stored by the body, so foods containing the vitamin should be eaten daily.

where to get it

Good sources include vegetables such as cabbage greens, red and yellow bell peppers, watercress, potatoes, peas, and snow peas; fruit such as oranges, strawberries, kiwi fruit, grapefruit, and other citrus fruits, black currants, mangoes, papayas, nectarines, peaches, raspberries, and tomatoes.

Vitamin C is destroyed by oxygen and heat, and it can also leach into water during cooking, so avoid overcooking its food sources.

Avoid smoking, stress, and fried foods, which prevent vitamin C from being absorbed and used by the body.

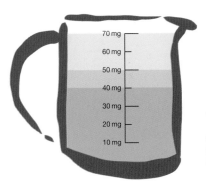

daily requirement of vitamin C

	normal daily requirement	60 mg
	during pregnancy	70 mg
	during lactation	70 mg

vitamin A retinol

Vitamin A is found in animal products; betacarotene is found in plant foods and converted by the body into vitamin A.

Vitamin A is essential for growth, healthy skin and hair, good vision, and healthy tooth enamel. Betacarotene is an important antioxidant essential for protection against heart disease and cancer, and as an immune booster. It is also needed for healthy skin and hair, and night vision.

why you need vitamin A during pregnancy

Vitamin A has antioxidant and protective properties which protect against damage to cells.

how much you need

The FDA recommends 4,000 IU (or 3 mg betacarotene). However, pregnant women or women who may become pregnant should avoid supplementation.

where to get it

Vitamin A is found in animal products as retinol (pre-formed vitamin A) and in plant foods as betacarotene, which the body can convert to vitamin A.

Sources of vitamin A (retinol) include liver and liver products, such as pâté (but see page 70), oily fish,

such as herring, mackerel, and trout, fish liver oils, milk, cheese, and margarine

and egg yolks. Foods rich in betacarotene include: carrots; dark green, leafy vegetables such as spinach, broccoli, cabbage, kale, Brussels sprouts, and watercress; asparagus; peas; beans; zucchini; leeks; lettuce; tomatoes; sweet potatoes; pumpkins; apricots; peaches (fresh and dried); mangoes; passion fruit; papayas; plums; watermelons;

and yellow-fleshed melons. Too much vitamin A (in the form of retinol) from animal sources can build up in the liver and cause damage to the fetus. However, this is extremely rare—you would need to eat a large quantity over a long period of time for this to be a problem (see page 70 for more information about vitamin A intake). Vegetable sources of vitamin A (betacarotene) don't cause any defects in an unborn child. (Ref. 2.12).

vitamin A source	vitamin A intake/source
8-oz smoked herring	74.25 ug
2 medium-sized eggs, scrambled	354.00 ug
½ cup plain strained yogurt	115.00 ug
1¾ oz Cheddar cheese	162.50 ug
3½ tbsp cream cheese	192.50 ug
2½ cups skim milk	312.40 ug

betacarotene source	betacarotene intake/source
12-oz (whole) papaya	2,835 ug
1½ cups mango	4,050 ug
3⅔ cups spinach, raw	3,888 ug
1½ cups sweet potatoes	4,356 ug
7-oz (whole medium) red bell pepper	7,560 ug
9½-inch carrot, raw and unpeeled	8,115 ug

vitamin D

Vitamin D, also known as cholecalciferol, works with calcium. Both are essential for normal growth and the growth and maintenance of healthy bones and teeth.

why you need vitamin D during pregnancy

Vitamin D supports fetal growth, the calcification (or the addition of calcium) of bone, and tooth and enamel formation.

how much you need

Vitamin D is obtained from sunlight but the FDA recommends 200 IU (5 mcg) for adults on a daily basis. However, research indicates that an unborn baby may suffer rather than the mother if she becomes deficient in this vitamin. A supplement may be required to achieve that amount.

where to get it

Vitamin D is made by the skin in the presence of sunlight. If you go outside every day, you are capable of synthesizing enough vitamin D from April to October to satisfy needs during those months and to build up liver stores to last through the remainder of the year. In addition, good food sources include seaweed; oily fish such as tuna, mackerel, smoked herring, canned sardines, and canned or fresh salmon; cod liver oil; liver (but *see* page 70); eggs; butter, and margarine; cheese; milk or soy drinks fortified with vitamin D; yogurt; and cereal fortified with vitamin D.

Vitamins A, C, and E help to protect vitamin D. Fried foods and a lack of sunlight work against it.

vitamin D source	vitamin D intake/source
⅓ cup sardines, canned	3.75 ug
8-oz smoked herring	56.25 ug
½ large can (7¼ oz) of salmon	26.25 ug
½ cup tuna in brine	2.60 ug
2 medium-sized eggs, scrambled	1.86 ug
1¾ oz Cheddar cheese	0.13 ug

vitamin E

Vitamin E, an antioxidant vitamin, helps develop and maintain strong cells, especially in the blood.

why you need vitamin E during pregnancy
General health requirements.

how much you need
The FDA recommends 12 IU (8 mg) for adult women and 15 IU (10 mg) for pregnant or nursing women.

where to get it
Good sources include avocados, mangoes, tomatoes, sweet potatoes, green, leafy vegetables (spinach, watercress, and lettuce), nuts, seeds, wheat germ, whole-grain cereals, milk, egg yolks, soft margarine, vegetable oils, sardines, and salmon.

vitamin E source	vitamin E intake/source
1 tbsp sunflower seeds	7.6 mg
2 tbsp hazelnuts	5.0 mg
2 tbsp almonds	4.8 mg
1 tbsp pine nuts	2.7 mg
1 tbsp peanuts	2.0 mg
whole medium-sized avocado	6.4 mg
1 tbsp sunflower oil	9.8 mg

supplements

In theory, if you eat a well-balanced (see pages 34–5) and healthy diet, you should not need supplements. However, the US FDA recommends that all women who are trying to conceive or who could be pregnant should take a daily supplement of 400 mcg of folic acid.

It also suggested that pregnant women need 5 mcg more than other adults. Any other decisions on whether to take a supplement are up to each individual but do seek medical advice.

There is no doubt that vitamin and mineral supplements have a valuable role to play, both in the prevention and treatment of a wide variety of health problems. However, pills are artificially manufactured, and there is growing evidence that naturally derived vitamins and minerals in food are more effective than those that are synthetically manufactured.

Nutrients in food are more easily absorbed by the body. It is therefore the advice of many experts that you eat a good varied diet to obtain all the essential nutrients you need from your food.

pregnancy & food safety

foods & safety

The immune system does not function as well as usual during pregnancy, so women are far more susceptible to the germs responsible for food poisoning.

safety in the home

Taking care in preparing food is very important if you are to avoid food poisoning. This is highly advisable, particularly during the first stages of pregnancy, because the immune system of an unborn baby is not sufficiently well-developed to fight infection.

general tips on food safety

- Wash your hands before and after handling food, especially when touching raw or cooked poultry and meat.
- Keep food surfaces in the kitchen clean and keep pets away from all food preparation areas.
- Use separate boards for preparing raw and cooked poultry and meat.
- Wash all boards thoroughly after using them.
- Don't eat food that has gone past its "use-by" date.
- Cook all food thoroughly, especially eggs, poultry, and meat.
- When reheating food, make sure it is piping hot all the way through.
- Wash all fruit and vegetables.
- Store eggs away from other foods as their shells may carry harmful bacteria. Also wash your hands after handling eggs.

fridge

● Keep your fridge between 32° and 39°F.

● Keep raw food on the bottom shelf of the fridge, so that if for any reason it leaks, it will not drip onto other foods. Keep raw food away from any cooked food.

● Wrap raw poultry and meat well to prevent them from dripping or leaking onto other foods.

pets

● Pets and other animals can pass on harmful bacteria that may be present in their feces. If these bacteria or other organisms are passed into your mouth, you can become infected with the bacteria, so after handling pets and animals it is important not to touch your mouth and to always wash your hands before eating or preparing food.

● Cat litter boxes need to be kept clean. If you have to clean them always wear rubber gloves, and wash your gloved hands, then your bare hands, thoroughly afterward.

● Also wear rubber gloves when gardening to protect your hands from toxoplasma, which may be present in the garden soil. Washing your hands after gardening is also prudent even if you have worn gloves.

● Sheep may miscarry or give birth to sick lambs following an infection, so don't help with lambing, handle newborn lambs, or come into close contact with sheep that have just given birth or miscarried. Boots and clothing that may be contaminated should not be brought into the house, but they should be cleaned thoroughly by someone else outside the house.

A blood test can determine whether or not you have listeriosis. Contact the doctor if symptoms develop (see below). A course of antibiotics can often prevent fetal infections.

safety in the diet

It is suspected that the immune system may not function as well as usual during pregnancy so women may be more susceptible to the germs responsible for food poisoning. Infections caused by contact with infected food or animals include the following.

listeria

Listeria bacteria can cause an illness known as listeriosis. This can feel like mild flu, with aches and pains, sore throat, and high temperatures. In rare circumstances it can progress into a more serious condition, causing septicemia (blood poisoning) and meningitis in newborn babies.

However, in some people the symptoms are so slight that they may not even be aware that they have had the illness. During pregnancy, listeria can be a problem since it can be passed from a mother to her unborn baby.

Although infection is rare, it is obviously sensible to avoid foods that are major sources of the listeria bacteria (see the rest of this chapter for more information) both before and during pregnancy.

Pregnant women are 20 times more likely than other healthy adults to get listeriosis.

Symptoms of infection can develop from two to 30 days after eating contaminated food.

Salmonella is one of the most common causes of food poisoning. It rarely causes damage to an unborn baby... but it is best to avoid any stress to your unborn child.

salmonella

Salmonella is one of the most common causes of food poisoning. It rarely causes damage to an unborn baby since the bacterium does not normally cross the placenta, but it is best to avoid salmonella to maintain good health and avoid any stress to your unborn child. Symptoms of this food poisoning include vomiting, diarrhea, very high temperatures, and dehydration. If you have salmonella, drink lots of fluids to replace lost liquids.

toxoplasmosis

This infection is caused by a parasite. It is not usually dangerous and may even go unnoticed in the healthy adult or unborn baby with just flu-like symptoms. However, in rare incidences toxoplasmosis has affected the health of the mother and/or the baby.

If you have had toxoplasmosis, you will be immune for life—a blood test can identify whether or not you are immune. If concerned, ask your doctor for such a test before you become pregnant.

The most common source of the bacteria may be found in animals' feces, specifically that of cats. Sensible hygiene precautions should be followed. Eating raw or uncooked meat or contact with infected soil can also pass on the disease.

cheese

what to avoid

The following cheeses can carry potentially dangerous bacteria called *Listeria monocytogenes*, although cases of listeria infection are rare.

Avoid all soft, semisoft, and blue cheeses. To be more specific, it is best to avoid both pasteurized and unpasteurized soft cheeses which usually have a surface mold and edible rind—for example, Brie, Camembert, feta, Montrachet, Neufchâtel, and Pont l'Evêque.

It is also best to avoid slightly more solid cheeses that do not grate easily and that are often coated with wax to preserve moisture and extend shelf life, such as Asiago, Belle Passe, Havarti, Muenster, Port-Salut, and Taleggio. Also stay away from the more solid blue cheeses, such as Stilton, Gorgonzola, and Roquefort.

what to eat

The UK's Department of Health says that the following cheeses are safe to eat: hard cheeses, e.g. cheddar, Parmesan; softer cheeses that do not have any mold or rind and are made from pasteurized milk, e.g. cottage cheese, ricotta, and mozzarella; processed cheese and cheese spreads.

Sometimes it is not easy to tell the type of cheese, so it is best to check the label. If you are not sure, play it safe and don't eat it.

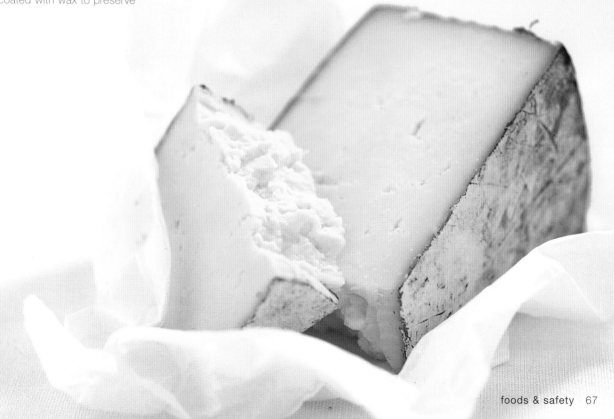

milk & cream

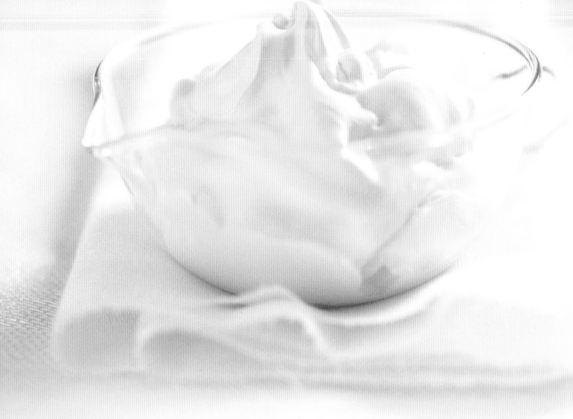

It is best to avoid
raw milk from
the time that you
start planning to
have a baby...

what to avoid

Health experts advise avoiding all
"raw" milk and cream from cows,
sheep, or goats. Raw milk has not
been pasteurized and may contain
bacteria and other organisms which
can cause illness. In particular,
unpasteurized goat's and sheep's
milk may contain the parasite
Toxoplasma gondii.

It is best to avoid raw milk from
the time that you start planning to
have baby to the time that you finish
breastfeeding.

what to eat

Pasteurized milk and cream are
readily available and are perfectly
safe, whether they come from cows,
sheep, or goats.

eggs

It is advisable to choose organic eggs, since their production requires a more stringently controlled food production system which has a high standard of hygiene.

what to avoid

The salmonella bacteria are most likely to be passed on through contaminated poultry and eggs. This applies to all types of eggs, whether they are duck, quail, or goose, etc. Even in some developed countries approximately one egg in every 450 is contaminated with salmonella.

It is advisable to choose organic eggs, since their production requires a more stringently controlled food production system which has a high standard of hygiene.

Avoid eating foods that contain raw or partly cooked egg, for example, mousse, homemade mayonnaise, sorbets, soft meringues, icing, and cheesecakes.

what to eat

The good news is that thorough cooking often eliminates salmonella, so it is fine to eat eggs that have been cooked so thoroughly that the egg yolks are hard. If you need to make a recipe that normally uses raw egg, try replacing the raw egg with pasteurized egg products which are available in supermarkets – pasteurization heats the eggs and kills the bacteria. While homemade mayonnaise should not be eaten, mayonnaise purchased in a grocery store is often safe to eat as long as it is made with pasteurized eggs, so check the label.

meat

raw or rare meats: what to avoid

Undercooked and raw poultry and meat may be contaminated with bacteria, which can cause food poisoning. These bacteria are destroyed when you cook food at high temperatures. Raw meat may also contain toxoplasma (see page 66), an organism which can, in rare cases, affect an unborn child.

It is also best to avoid foods preserved in nitrates, such as smoked or cured meats, frankfurters, salami, and luncheon meats (Ref. 3.1).

what to eat

The UK's Department of Health advises cooking all meat and poultry, including burgers and sausages, until the juices run clear and there is no remaining blood or pinkness. This is because any bacteria that may be present are destroyed when exposed to high temperatures.

Wash your hands thoroughly when handling raw meat and store raw foods separately from cooked foods.

liver: what to avoid

There is a risk to pregnant women of excessive intake of vitamin A in the form of retinol from liver and liver products. In recent years, the vitamin A content of animal liver has increased considerably, probably due to changes in feeding practices. A 3½-oz portion of liver can contain between 20,000–40,000 mcg of vitamin A, depending on the animal.

This is obviously unacceptably high when you consider that the upper safe level is 8,000 to 10,000 mcg per day for pregnant women. Nutritional experts therefore recommend that women who are trying to become pregnant or who are pregnant should avoid eating liver and liver products such as pâté and liver sausage.

In addition, meat pâté may contain high levels of listeria.

Undercooked and raw poultry and meat may be contaminated with bacteria, which can cause food poisoning.

seafood & fish

what to avoid

Pregnant women are advised not to eat oysters. They are also advised to avoid shelled seafood such as shrimp, mussels, and crabs, unless they are a part of a hot meal and have been thoroughly cooked. When raw, these foods may be contaminated with harmful bacteria and viruses.

It is also recommended that pregnant women limit their intakes of predatory fish such as swordfish, fresh tuna, and shark—all of which are mercury-rich—to no more than one serving per month. However, levels of mercury in canned tuna are lower, so it is fine to eat a couple of cans per week.

Do not eat fish from contaminated waters or tropical fish such as grouper, amberjack, and mahi-mahi. It is also best to avoid foods preserved in nitrates—for example, smoked fish.

what to eat

Because unwanted chemicals collect in fatty tissue, it is best to eat lean seafood such as sole, flounder, haddock, Pacific halibut, ocean perch, pollack, and cod. Salmon is also fine. Seafood should be well cooked.

Most fresh fish from reputable suppliers and restaurants are safe to eat during pregnancy.

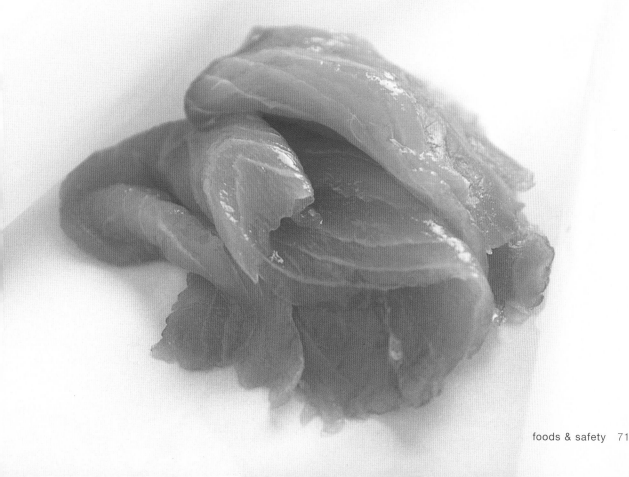

salads

...avoid ready-made dressed salads, such as potato salad and coleslaw...

what to avoid

Pre-packaged salads—available in bags from supermarkets—may contain listeria bacteria. You should also avoid ready-made dressed salads, such as potato salad and coleslaw for the same reasons. In addition, salad leaves that have not been thoroughly washed may carry the toxoplasmosis parasite (*see* page 66).

what to eat

Make your own salads. All salad ingredients should be washed well in order to remove any soil or dirt. It is also advisable to wash thoroughly any soil from your hands and kitchen surfaces.

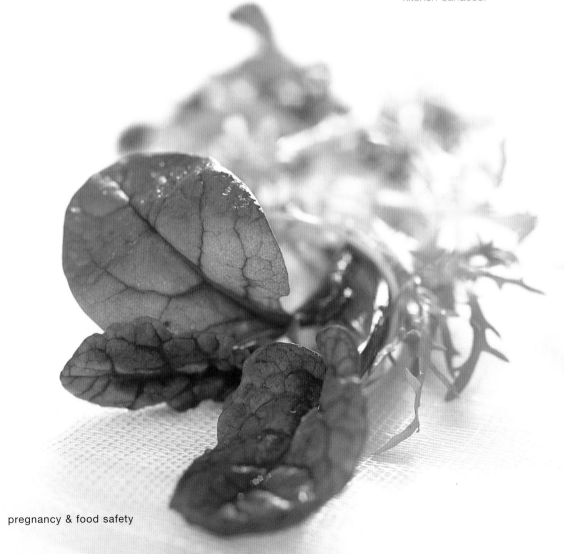

convenience foods

what to avoid

Raw or undercooked ready-prepared meals should be avoided due to the risk of listeria. This bacteria has been found in cooked-chilled meals and also in ready-to-eat poultry, including plain roast chicken. It is important to note that listeria bacteria can multiply even at low temperatures, such as inside a supermarket chill cabinet or your refrigerator.

what to eat

While ready-prepared meals can be eaten, they must be reheated until they are piping hot throughout.

The following guidelines can help you store and cook foods properly.

● Whenever possible, keep chilled convenience foods cool, preferably in an insulated bag or box during travel and transfer them straight to the fridge.

● Keep your fridge temperature between 32° and 39°F.

● Always eat foods by their "best-before" date; this way, any bacteria that the foods do contain may not have multiplied to dangerous levels.

● Follow instructions on reheating the foods carefully. Because listeria bacteria are not killed by low temperatures, thorough reheating is essential. If you are using an oven, allow time for it to preheat. If you are using a microwave, check that you are using the cooking times appropriate to the microwave's power level. Always follow instructions about standing times or stirring; this helps to distribute the heat evenly.

● Before eating food, check that the middle is piping hot.

Follow instructions on reheating the foods carefully. Because listeria bacteria are not killed by low temperatures, thorough reheating is essential.

nuts

...exclusive breastfeeding for the first six months helps decrease the risk of allergies in our baby's early years.

what to avoid

Avoid peanuts if you, your baby's father, or one of your previous children suffers from any allergic conditions. These include eczema, asthma, allergic rhinitis (hay fever), and any allergic response (rashes, itches, and bumps) after eating food such as strawberries, shellfish, or peanuts.

Peanut allergy is a growing problem. Approximately one in 200 four-year-old children has a peanut allergy; most of these children will develop the problem before their third birthday. In rare cases, peanut allergy can cause a severe reaction called anaphylactic shock, which can be life-threatening.

Before an allergy can develop, a child first has to come into contact with small traces of peanut. This initial contact can cause a future reaction when the child eats peanuts or foods containing peanuts. Some experts now think that this initial sensitization may occur during pregnancy, when a tiny amount of the peanut protein crosses the placenta. There is no definitive evidence to prove this yet, and further research is needed. However, because peanut allergy is an increasing problem, it has been advised that women with an allergic reaction to peanuts or women who know of a family member that has an allergic reaction to peanuts should avoid them while pregnant or breastfeeding.

Breastfeeding gives your baby protection against many infections; exclusive breastfeeding for the first six months helps decrease the risk of allergies in your baby's early years. However, if you eat peanuts, there is a small chance that your baby will come into contact with traces of peanut through your milk.

As stated above, if you decide to avoid peanuts while pregnant or breastfeeding, you need to avoid not only peanuts themselves—which are also sometimes called groundnuts, or goober peas in the South—but also any products that may contain them. These include peanut butter, cereals, cakes, granola, cookies, some salad dressings, ice cream, and breads.

Always read the packaging label carefully for information on ingredients. Supermarkets should be able to provide a list of the nut-free products it produces and sells.

When ordering dishes in restaurants, either ask if peanuts have been included or choose a simple meal which contains no "hidden" ingredients.

what to eat

For everyone else, nuts and seeds are a great source of protein, fat, B vitamins, and iron. Because they are so high in fat, they also tend to be high in calories, so it is worth bearing this in mind when you eat them as a snack.

...nuts and seeds are a great source of protein, fat, B vitamins, and iron.

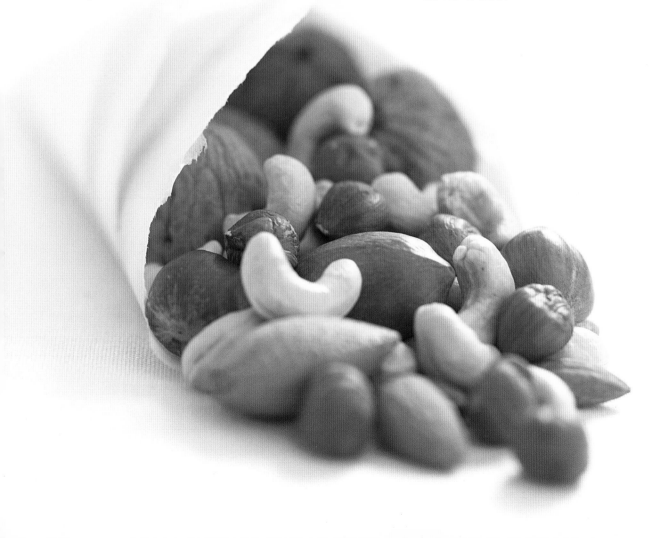

foods & comfort

nausea & sickness

Try drinking rice water. Take small sips of the warm water left in the saucepan after you have boiled rice.

what it is

Morning sickness, which tends to affect seven in 10 women, is a feeling of nausea and, in some cases, vomiting, which often occurs in the morning but can happen at any time during the day. It is caused by hormonal and metabolic changes and usually lasts no longer than the first three months. However, some women can spend their whole nine months feeling sick and throwing up. If you go for more than a day without being able to keep anything down, it is a good idea to visit your doctor or dietician.

how to avoid it

Some of the following suggestions may work for you.

● Use fresh ginger root—known to help relieve nause—in cooking, or drink ginger tea.

● Peppermint, ginger, and camomile herbal teas are also very soothing.

● Some carbonated drinks, for example, ginger ale, are also good for relieving nausea.

● Try drinking rice water. Take small sips of the warm water left in the saucepan after you have boiled rice.

● Try to eat something, such as crackers, plain toast, dry cereal, or anything else that may appeal before getting out of bed in the morning. This will help keep blood-sugar levels steady. Resist chocolate, buttery, or creamy cookies and pastries, since these often aggravate nausea.

• An empty stomach can make nausea worse, so don't go for long periods without eating; eat frequent small meals or snacks. Fruit and seeds make great snacks. *See* pages 126–31 for more snack ideas.

• Try to avoid high-fat and fried foods, which are particularly difficult to digest. Starchy foods such as bread, pasta, rice, and potatoes are far gentler on the system.

• Make sure your diet is as varied and balanced as possible. One school of thought maintains that morning sickness only occurs in women whose nutrition is less than optimum (*Ref. 3.2*).

• One possible explanation for morning sickness is that the body is trying to get rid of toxins.

• Women low in B_6 and zinc may have a higher risk of suffering from morning sickness (*Ref. 3.3*). *See* page 55 for foods containing vitamin B_6.

• Avoid all sugar, refined foods, and high-fat junk food which contain large quantities of additives and preservatives.

• Drink lots of water between meals.
• Decrease consumption of coffee and tea. They can aggravate nausea and vomiting.
• Avoid alcohol and cigarettes.
• Avoid strong smells.
• Try to get some fresh air prior to eating. If you have the time, a quick stroll before food is a good idea.

supplements

According to Dr. Pfeiffer and Nim Barnes of the Foresight Association (*see* page 9), "The nauseated woman is usually deficient in both zinc and B_6. Both are needed for growing tissues of any kind, and the fetus and uterus make extraordinary demands on the mother's supply. We have had many pregnant patients who had difficulties with previous pregnancies go through a pregnancy on a zinc and B_6 regime with no difficulties."

If nausea and sickness persist it may be worthwhile getting your doctor to check your nutritional status to assess if further supplementation is necessary.

One possible explanation for morning sickness is that the body is trying to get rid of toxins.

weight

It is advised that you lose excess weight well in advance of your planned pregnancy...

It is possible that your pre-pregnancy weight can have a direct impact on the birth weight of your baby.

Body Mass Index, or BMI, is an index of a person's weight in relation to height. It is calculated by dividing your weight (in kilograms) by the square of your height (in meters): $BMI = kg/m^2$

Weight in pounds can be converted to kilograms by multiplying pounds by 0.4536. Height in inches can be converted to meters by multiplying inches by 0.0254. A BMI of 23 to 24 is considered good for general health, fertility, and birth weight (Ref. 3.5).

underweight

If you have a low BMI, this may also be an indication of a poor nutritional status, which is linked to low birth weight. A study of underweight women and pregnancy outcome showed that underweight women (BMI below 19.1 kg/m²) had a three-fold increased risk of having a baby with a low birth weight.

overweight

Women who are overweight when they conceive (BMIs over 30) are more likely to face pregnancy problems such as hypertension, pre-eclampsia, and gestational diabetes. It is therefore advised to lose excess weight well in advance of your planned pregnancy, allowing at least two or three months of good, well-balanced nutrition before conception. It is not advised to attempt to diet when pregnant.

normal Body Mass Index (BMI) gradations

	BMI
Underweight	less than 20
Acceptable weight	20–24.9
Overweight	25–29.9
Fat	30–39.9
Very fat	greater than 40

weight gain

How much you gain during your pregnancy depends on your height and how much you weighed before you conceived. If you were underweight, you are likely to gain between 28 lb and 39 lb; if you were an average pre-pregnancy weight, you should gain between 24 lb and 35 lb; and if you were overweight, between 15 lb and 24 lb. If you are having twins, the average weight gain is about 35 lb to 44 lb. (*Ref. 3.6*).

The increased blood volume, breast and uterine tissue, amniotic fluid, baby, placenta, and fluid retention—all products of pregnancy—account for about 10 lb to 15 lb of normal pregnancy weight gain. Women who are overweight may find that they only gain a small amount as their bodies intuitively know that they do not need extra fat storage (*Ref. 3.7*).

If you are concerned that you are not gaining enough weight, try the following suggestions.
- Eat small meals often.
- Try to ensure that the meals are as full of energy as possible. Make sure that your diet consists of a variety of protein, carbohydrates, and good fats.
- Also eat nutrient-rich foods such as cheese, milk, yogurt made with whole milk, fish, cream, meat, and butter. Dried fruits, such as apricots, figs, and prunes, are good foods to snack on.

If you are concerned that you are gaining too much weight too soon, reduce the number of calories you eat and concentrate on eating nutrient-rich foods.
- When cooking, use a minimum amount of fat.
- Snack on fresh, poached, or dried fruit, either on its own or with some ricotta cheese or yogurt.
- *See* the recommended guide to healthy eating (page 35).

Women who are overweight may find that they only gain a small amount as their bodies intuitively know that they do not need extra fat storage.

indigestion

what it is

Heartburn is very common in the later stages of pregnancy. This can be caused partly by the baby's body pressing on your stomach. Also, the hormone changes during pregnancy can cause the muscles at the top of your stomach to over-relax, making it more likely that its acidic contents will leak into your esophagus. The presence of these acidic juices in your esophagus causes an acidic, unpleasant sensation—heartburn. This complaint is often made worse at night, when you are lying down.

how to avoid it

● It is important not to rely on medication, which can interfere with absorption of vitamins and minerals.
● Avoid large meals. Choose small, frequent meals or snacks instead.
● Avoid eating fatty foods on an empty stomach. Also avoid foods that you find hard to digest.
● Take time when eating, and chew food properly.
● Sit up straight when eating and avoid activity just after a meal.
● Carbonated drinks, citrus fruits, soda, caffeine, alcohol, processed meats, and spicy, highly seasoned, fried fatty foods can make the problem worse.
● Avoid drinking too much when you are eating.
● Try to gain a sensible amount of weight (see page 79).
● Do not eat too late at night.
● Sleep with your head propped up a little.
● Sip settling drinks such as peppermint or ginger tea, or ice water.
● Some experts advise avoiding antacid preparations, unless recommended by your doctor, healthcare practitioner, or pharmacist. Some of these contain high levels of aluminum or sodium, which are not ideal for pregnant women.

It is important not to rely on medication, which can interfere with absorption of vitamins and minerals.

cravings

what they are

Cravings usually occur in the first and last three months of pregnancy, when the body experiences dramatic changes. Some women experience cravings for the strangest foods—about 85 per cent of women report at least one food craving during pregnancy. American Babycenter.com users confessed to wanting pickles wrapped in cheese, salsa spooned straight out of the jar, and even steak fat (*Ref. 3.10*). "Quite a lot of cravings are for out-of-season foods and foods which bear no resemblance to things previously liked by women," says Cornian Casey-Hardman, a senior midwife at The Liverpool Women's Hospital (*Ref. 3.11*). Usually such cravings are not a problem, as long as you are still able to eat a well-balanced diet. You may also experience strong aversions to fatty foods, alcohol, tea, and coffee.

Cravings can be interpreted in several ways. Later on in pregnancy, some women develop cravings for hot, spicy food. This can be because their senses of taste has reduced, so they crave more highly flavored foods.

...about 85 per cent of women report at least one food craving...

There is also some evidence that particularly strange cravings for substances such as coal are due to a lack of certain key nutrients in the system, while others may be due to comfort eating.

A possible explanation for cravings is a change in taste and smell during pregnancy. Cravings may be caused by an impaired sense of taste, while aversions are more likely to be due to an altered sense of smell.

Some cravings and aversions can arise subconsciously if you are trying to improve your diet and avoid unhealthy food and drink.

There is also research that indicates that hormonal changes can cause cravings. This has also been shown in nonfood cravings such as smells or an increased desire for sex.

constipation & hemorrhoids

what they are

Constipation can occur when extra hormones produced in pregnancy cause the intestine to relax and become less efficient. Coupled with pressure from the baby, this can, over time, lead to the development of hemorrhoids (varicose veins of the anus). Sometimes hemorrhoids only appear for the first time during labor as you strain to push your baby out. Luckily, pregnancy hemorrhoids nearly always disappear within three months of giving birth.

Another reason that pregnancy also makes women more prone to hemorrhoids—and, similarly, to bleeding gums—is because the amount of blood circulating through your body increases. This causes all your veins to become dilated. In particular, the veins below the level of your uterus are susceptible to becoming varicose—abnormally swollen or dilated—as the uterus places increased pressure on them.

how to avoid them

● Eat plenty of fresh fruit, vegetables,and whole-grain cereals.
● Eat dried fruit.
● Drink lots of water—at least three and a half pints a day.
● Swimming and other light exercise can also help.

Sometimes hemorrhoids only appear for the first time during labor ... pregnancy hemorrhoids nearly always disappear within three months of giving birth.

anemia

what it is

A mild form of anemia may be present in one in three pregnant women. Symptoms include pallor, tiredness, a sore tongue, unusual tiredness, and feeling as if the weight of the world is on your shoulders (*Ref. 3.12*).

how to avoid it

Anemia is usually the result of a low level of iron, although vitamin B_{12}, folic acid, manganese, and vitamin B_6 deficiency can also contribute (*see* the section on iron, page 51).

insomnia

what it is

Not being able to sleep at night is something that almost all pregnant women experience at some point during the last few weeks of their pregnancies. This is hardly surprising—the size of your tummy makes it difficult to get comfortable, You may be getting up several times to go to the bathroom, your baby may be kicking, or you may be woken by cramps. You may also be kept awake by worry, or be woken by disturbing dreams.

Pregnant women barely sleep enough for one person, let alone two, according to the US National Sleep Foundation (NSF) 1998 Women and Sleep Poll (WSP). A whopping 79 per cent of women who took part in the poll said their sleep is more disturbed during pregnancy than at other times.

The study states that many pregnant women make up for their sleep deficits by napping—they are almost twice as likely to be sleepy during the day than other women. Half of pregnant or recently pregnant women—51 per cent—take at least one weekday nap, and 60 per cent take at least one nap on weekends.

how to avoid it

- Lie on your side with a pillow under your bump and another between your knees.
- Practice relaxation exercises, particularly breathing slowly and deeply when trying to get to sleep.
- Have a warm bath before going to bed.
- Have a warm, milky drink before going to bed.
- Have a massage at bedtime.
- Do some gentle exercise— for example, walking or swimming— during the day.
- Just as with any significant problems in sleeping, rest as much as possible during the day to make up for the sleep lost at night.

Have a warm, milky drink before going to bed.

cramps

what they are

Cramps are very likely to be caused by an imbalance of calcium and magnesium. Other possible causes of pregnancy-related leg cramps include the following:

- an excess of phosphorus and a shortage of calcium circulating in the blood;
- the pressure of the expanding uterus on the nerves leading to the legs;
- decreased circulation in the legs from the pressure of the baby on blood vessels;
- tired muscles. The extra weight on your leg muscles can lead to night cramps, which can wake you out of a sound sleep. Leg cramps normally occur between three and nine months of pregnancy (*Ref. 3.13*).

Other possible causes of pregnancy-related leg cramps include... an excess of phosphorus and a shortage of calcium circulating in the blood.

how to avoid them

If you find yourself with cramps, try the following steps to relieve the pain.

- Walk. This may be uncomfortable at first, but it helps relieve cramps.
- Stand with your legs straight and bend your toes toward your head, without bending your knees.
- Try resting with your legs raised on pillows or the arm of a sofa.
- Avoid massaging your legs if they have red or especially painful spots.
- Stretching your calf muscles several times before going to bed can help.
- Avoid standing for long periods or sitting with your legs crossed.
- Eat calcium-rich foods.
- Avoid soft drinks—they contain a lot of phosphorus.
- Moderate exercise may help.
- Avoid wearing constrictive clothing of any type.
- Wear shoes with low heels.
- Rest, especially if standing for long hours during the day.

drugs & safety

hot drinks

caffeine

Research is inconsistent about the effects of drinking more than five cups of coffee a day, which is why experts don't always agree on how to advise pregnant women. My advice would be to drink up to one or two cups of coffee or equivalent a day, and if possible, to cut it out completely. Decaffeinated drinks are not recommended as they can contain other stimulants and possibly harmful residues, such as pesticides (*Ref. 3.14*).

A mug of instant coffee contains 100 mg of caffeine, a mug of ground coffee up to 150 mg, and a mug of tea between 80 and 100 mg. The substance is also present in cola-based drinks, chocolate, and cocoa.

The effects of caffeine during pregnancy are not fully known. However, many experts believe that ingesting too much caffeine may contribute to the risk of babies being born with a low birth weight.

The *Journal of the American Medical Association* reported a study which found that the risk of miscarriage doubled in women who drank two or three cups of ground coffee or its equivalent daily (*Ref. 3.15*).

Other studies have linked miscarriage, low birth weight, and birth defects to large amounts of caffeine. However, much of this research failed to take into account other risk factors such as smoking and alcohol intake, which can also lead to complications in pregnancy, labor, and delivery.

Caffeine is a stimulant; it increases your heart rate and metabolism, which in turn affects your developing baby. But while constant stress is not healthy, brief bouts of fetal stress, such as that your baby would feel after you've drunk a cup of coffee, won't cause him or her any harm—it briefly boosts your heart rate and metabolism.

Caffeine is also a diuretic, and it can interfere with the absorption of certain nutrients.

what to avoid

Coffee, tea, sodas, and chocolate in large quantities. Some over-the-counter drugs including headache and cold tablets, stay-awake medications, and allergy remedies may also contain caffeine. If you are consuming a lot of caffeine daily, it is best to wean yourself off the substance gradually.

herbal teas

Look on packaging labels for contents that may normally be part of your diet, such as mint or orange extracts. Choose them over unfamiliar substances such as black cohosh root or mugwort.

alcohol

Professor Matthew Kaufman, an expert on early embryology, says of alcohol: "The only thing we can say is [that] 'safe' is none at all until child-bearing is over." This is supported by the Surgeon General of the United States: "Pregnant women and those planning a pregnancy should abstain from the use of alcohol."

Experts are not able to say how much or how little alcohol can harm a developing baby. Danger levels are most likely different for each individual woman because everyone metabolizes alcohol differently. It is felt that the effects of alcohol are greater in women who smoke, consume large amounts of caffeine, and have a poor diet.

Some health bodies, including the recommend that pregnant women play it safe by steering clear of alcohol completely. Others, such as the

recommend that women should simply limit their intake to one unit of alcohol per day (half a pint of beer, a glass of wine, a small glass of sherry, or a single measure of spirits).

It is stgonrly recommended by medical to minimize risk to unborn children, pregnant women should drink no more than one or two units of alcohol once or twice a week, and should avoid heavy drinking sessions.

Foresight (see page 9) takes the view that both partners should abstain from alcohol in the preconception phase, and that women should continue to stay away from alcohol throughout pregnancy (see page 29 for more information on fertility and alcohol).

The World Health Organization, says: "No alcohol during pregnancy is the only safe limit."

what to do and why

Toxins from alcohol are at their most dangerous during the first few weeks of pregnancy, so it is a good idea to stop drinking alcohol at least two weeks before conception.

It is thought that alcohol crosses the placenta freely and babies receive the alcohol before it is broken down by the mother's liver. A baby's own liver only starts forming some four weeks after conception and cannot deal with the alcohol, so damage may occur (Ref. 3.16).

Alcohol is sometimes described as an "anti-nutrient" because its consumption can lead to malabsorption, or increased urinary excretion of nutrients needed during pregnancy—in particular, thiamine, zinc, vitamin A, and folic acid. ·

However, if you have discovered that you are pregnant and you have been drinking, try not to worry. A great many women have had a drink or two before they knew they were pregnant and their babies have been fine.

proven risks

Women who drink over six units of alcohol per day are at risk of having babies with fetal alcohol syndrome (FAS). Children born with FAS may suffer from mental and growth retardation, behavioral problems, and facial and heart defects.

Babies of women who drink more than two glasses of alcohol a day throughout their pregnancy are more likely to have problems with learning speech, attention span, language, and hyperactivity than babies of women who did not drink. These are known as Fetal Alcohol Effects (FAE).

nicotine

what to do and why

Many professional experts advise stopping smoking long before you try to conceive. If it is not possible to stop completely, it is advised that you cut down. This applies to both the mother- and father-to-be.

In the US, smoking during pregnancy has been identified as the single most important preventable determinant of low birth weight and perinatal death. As well as infertility (see page 30), other links that have been formed between smoking and pregnancy outcome include miscarriage, premature delivery, physical abnormalities at birth, and stillbirth (Ref. 3.17).

smoking and miscarriage

Expectant mothers who smoke may have lower levels of hormones, which has led researchers to believe that this could be one reason why smoking results in ill effects to unborn babies. Miscarriages are known to be influenced by hormonal changes.

smoking and birth weight

The higher the number of cigarettes smoked by the expectant mother, the lower the birth weight is likely to be. This effect on birth size is caused by the cigarette's ability to slow down the rate of growth of the fetus. It may do this by damaging the DNA. In turn, this has consequences for mental and physical development.

fathers and smoking

A large study in Germany has shown that even when only the father smokes, there is an increased incidence of pregnancy and birth problems (Ref. 3.19).

Although research has shown that multivitamin supplementation appears to offer some protection against the risk of low birth weight, it is strongly advisable simply to stop smoking altogether.

how to quit

The good news is that more people succeed in stopping smoking when planning to become pregnant or during pregnancy than at other times—women wish to stop because they want to give their babies the best possible chance while in their womb.

pregnancy recipes

three meals
a day

...if you eat small meals frequently, you are more likely to feel good, keep your energy levels constant, and eat a greater variety of nutrients throughout the day...

I have developed recipes for breakfasts, lunches, suppers, and snacks that rely heavily on fresh fruit, vegetables, and seeds. These recipe ideas are based around fresh fruits, vegetables, and stamina foods such as whole grains, legumes (beans, lentils etc) fish, and meat—all of which provide a variety of nutrients needed for a healthy pregnancy.

Breakfast is too important to miss. Studies show that if you eat a high-carbohydrate breakfast, it can result in a lower overall intake of fat throughout the day. By skipping breakfast, you are more likely to binge on high-fat foods later. Eat a good lunch that will not leave you feeling too full or heavy. Lunches high in carbohydrates are difficult for the system to digest and can put strain on the body, leaving you feeling tired. The lunches in this book are all relatively light, providing a good mix of protein, carbohydrates, and lots of vitamins and minerals.

Aim to eat supper a good few hours before going to bed so that your bodies have time to digest the food before you sleep.

I believe that if you eat small meals frequently you are more likely to feel good, keep your energy levels constant, and eat a greater variety of nutrients throughout the day. For this reason, I have developed a few snack recipes for you to try.

When it comes to choosing ingredients, go for fresh and, wherever possible, seasonal and organic. For information about organic foods, *see* pages 38-39.

breakfasts

smoothies

strawberry shake

Serves: 2

1⅓ cups strawberries

1 banana, peeled and chopped

fortified soy drink (milk alternative), enough to make a good consistency

a little sugar, to taste (optional)

Strawberries are a good source of **betacarotene**, which helps to boost the immune system. Bananas are a good source of **folic acid** and fortified soy drink provides **protein**.

1 Throw the fruit into a food processor or blender with a little soy drink and puree until smooth.

2 Add enough milk to make a smooth, thick (but not too thick) shake. Add sugar to taste.

mango & melon smoothie

Serves: 2

1 mango

½ melon, e.g. honeydew or muskmelon, peeled and seeded

sparkling water (optional)

A whole mango provides more than the daily requirement of **vitamin C**. Melons provide **folic acid**, which helps to prevent birth defects.

1 Cut the mango either side of the seed, peel the flesh, and put into a food processor or blender.

2 Add the melon flesh and puree until smooth. Add sparkling water if you want to dilute it slightly.

fiber-boost fruit smoothies

Serves: 2

1 cup skim milk or fortified soy drink

4 tbsp plain yogurt

2 tsp liquid honey

1 tbsp oat germ

1 tbsp wheat germ

fruit of your choice, e.g. 1 banana, peeled and chopped

or 1 banana, peeled and chopped, handful of raspberries, and handful of blueberries

or 1 banana, peeled and chopped, and 1 passion fruit, halved and flesh scooped out

or ½ mango, peeled and seeded, and 1 passion fruit, halved and flesh scooped out

or 6 dried apricots, chopped

Oat germ, wheat germ, and fruit are all great sources of soluble **fiber**, while the milk and yogurt provide **calcium** and **protein**. The fruit also gives your body a few **vitamins** and **minerals**.

1 Put the first five ingredients with one of the fruit combinations (*see left*) of your choice into a food processor or blender

2 Puree until smooth.

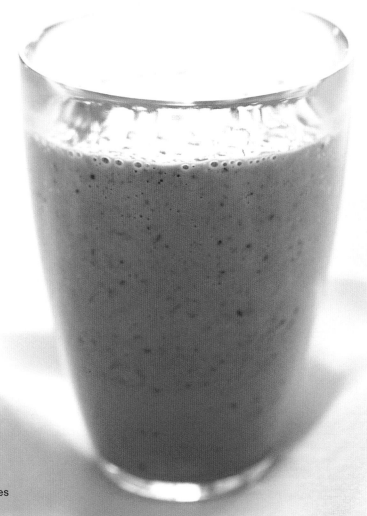

papaya, melon, & grape smoothie

Serves: 2–3 (halve the ingredients if you want to make one large drink)

2 papayas
½ muskmelon
juice of ½ lime
small bunch of seedless grapes
sparkling water

Papapya and muskmelon are excellent sources of **betacarotene**, which is essential for reproduction and growth. The bubbles in sparkling water can help to alleviate morning sickness.

1 Cut the papayas in half and scoop out the seeds. Peel and put the flesh into a food processor or blender. Scoop the seeds from the melon, peel, and add the melon flesh to the processor or blender.

2 Add the lime juice and grapes, and puree until smooth. You may need to add sparkling water to make the right consistency.

mango & banana smoothie

Serves: 2

½ mango
½ banana, peeled and chopped
juice of ½ lime
pinch of ground cardamom
1 cup plain yogurt
½ cup water
a little brown sugar or honey, to taste
ice cubes (optional)

The banana will supply a good source of energy, and the mango and lime will give you a burst of **vitamin C**, which will help to boost the immune system. Adding yogurt to a smoothie is a quick and easy way of incorporating **calcium** into the diet.

1 Slice the mango either side of the seed, peel one half, and put the flesh into a food processor or blender. Add the banana, lime juice, cardamom, yogurt, and water, and puree for about 30 seconds, until smooth.

2 Pour it into glasses and add sugar or honey to taste and ice cubes, if using.

(diluted with water)

citrus drink

Serves: 2

2 oranges
1 grapefruit
lime juice, to taste
ice cubes (optional)

Wake up with one of these. Oranges, grapefruit, and limes are an excellent source of **vitamin C**, while grapefruit contains pectin, which helps to lower cholesterol levels in the blood.

1 Cut the oranges and grapefruit in half and squeeze out all the juice.
2 Add lime juice to taste and ice cubes, if using. Drink and enjoy.

fruits

mango & strawberries with toasted oats

Serves: 2

⅓ cup organic rolled oats
1 large ripe mango, peeled, seeded, and chopped
6 strawberries, sliced
juice of ½ lime
½ cup strained, plain yogurt
honey, to taste

This is an easy way to incorporate more fresh fruit into your diet. Toasting the rolled oats gives them a wonderful crunch and they will help to keep your energy levels up during the morning.

1 Lightly toast the oats in a dry skillet until lightly golden. Toss the fruit with the lime juice and put into two dishes.

2 Top with yogurt and the toasted oats. Drizzle with honey.

vanilla roasted fruits

Serves: 4

2 lbs (about 14) plums
3 peaches or nectarines
1 vanilla pod
1–2 tbsp sugar, to taste

These fruits make a great change to fresh fruit, mixed with yogurt and cereal for breakfast. Alternatively, use to make into a crisp for supper. If the fruit is naturally sweet, add only a little sugar. Choose any fruit in season: plums, nectarines, figs, cherries, pears, and apples all work really well.

1 Preheat the oven to 400°F. Cut the plums and peaches or nectarines in half, remove the stones, and put the fruit into an ovenproof dish.
2 Cut a slit in the vanilla pod and scrape half the seeds into a bowl; add the sugar, and mix together. Scatter the vanilla sugar over the fruit and roast for approximately 10 minutes, until the fruit is slightly soft, but still holding its shape. Alternatively, put the fruit under a hot broiler for five minutes.
3 Serve with yogurt and cereal, or use as the base for a crisp.

dried fruit compote

Serves: 4

¾ cup apple juice

¾ cup orange juice

2 cups mixed dried fruit, e.g. pears, peaches, prunes, apricots, and figs

handful of raisins

½ tsp ground cinnamon and 1 cinnamon stick

Cooking the dried fruit in juice makes it really plump and sweet. Choose fruit that you like—I used pears, peaches, figs, etc. Alternatively, you could use a bag of mixed dried fruit. This will keep for a few days; cover and store in the fridge.

Mixed dried fruit is a good source of **iron** and **folic acid**. Apple and orange juice are both good sources of **vitamin C**, which improves iron absorption in the body.

1 Put all the ingredients into a saucepan and bring to a boil.

2 Remove from the heat and leave to cool.

fresh fruit salad with raspberry sauce

Serves: 2

a selection of fresh fruit of your choice, e.g. 1 each mango or nectarine and papaya, prepared and cut into chunks

for the raspberry sauce:

1 cup frozen or fresh raspberries or mixed berries

1–2 tsp sugar

squeeze of lime or lemon juice

yogurt and sunflower seeds, to serve

Fresh fruit is a good source of **fiber** and **vitamin C**, which helps the body with digestion and absorption of iron. Yogurt provides **calcium**, which helps with the formation of bones.

Another delicious winning combination is a mixture of melon, papaya, and fresh basil or mint, with a little maple syrup drizzled over the top.

1 Make the sauce; put all the ingredients in a heavy saucepan and simmer until the raspberries have turned to a pulp. Taste for sweetness; leave to cool.

2 Scatter your chosen fresh fruit over two plates and drizzle the raspberry sauce over the top, finishing with a dollop of yogurt and a sprinkling of sunflower seeds.

cereals

nutty fruity bar

Makes: 15

3 tbsp butter

2 tbsp sugar

⅓ cup light corn syrup

1⅔ cups jumbo rolled oats

¼ cup pumpkin seeds, toasted

⅓ cup Brazil nuts, chopped and toasted

⅓ cup dried apricots, roughly chopped

⅓ cup dried mango, cut into small pieces

1 tbsp sesame seeds, toasted

Once you have made these, you can just grab one as and when you choose. They will keep in an airtight container or in the freezer.

These bars are packed with goodness; the oats provide **folic acid**, and the seeds and nuts are good sources of **zinc**, **calcium**, and **iron**.

1 Grease an 8-inch square pan. Preheat the oven to 350°F. Put the butter, sugar, and syrup into a saucepan and heat until the butter has melted.

2 Add all the other ingredients and mix well. Tip into the greased pan and bake in the oven for 25–30 minutes.

3 Mark into squares and leave to cool in the tin. Cut and store in an airtight container.

creamy porridge

Serves: 4

1½ cups milk

1½ cups water

1 cup organic oatmeal

topping suggestions:

a selection of fresh fruit, chopped into pieces

a couple of spoons of Dried Fruit Compote (page 95) or Vanilla Roasted Fruits (page 94)

chopped banana and dates with a little molasses

a sprinkling of wheat germ and a chopped kiwi fruit with a drizzle of honey

dark Barbados sugar or molasses sugar

I find porridge one of the best ways to start the day. The oats provide slow-release energy and **B-complex vitamins**, keeping your energy levels constant through the morning. Always add some soy drink or milk for **protein** and pile fresh or dried fruit on top—whatever is handy. Traditionally, a little pinch of salt is added, but I prefer it without.

1 Put the milk and water into a saucepan and add the oats. Bring to a boil, reduce to a simmer, and cook for five minutes.

2 Serve the porridge with any one of the suggested toppings.

dried fruit & nut granola

Makes: 6–8

⅓ cup sunflower seeds

⅓ cup almonds, roughly chopped

½ cup whole hazelnuts or cashews, roughly chopped

⅔ cup coconut chips (available from supermarkets) or desiccated coconut

2 cup rolled oats

4 tbsp wheat germ

⅔ cup each dried apricots, chopped, and raisins

½ cup dried cranberries or blueberries

pinch of freshly grated or ground nutmeg

½ tsp cinnamon

choose milk; soy drink; plain or soy yogurt; fruit juice and fresh fruit, to serve

This is easy and quick to make, and will last for a good few breakfasts; just keep it in an airtight jar. To make the granola toddler- or baby-friendly, puree in a food processor to a powder. However, avoid giving it to babies or toddlers with nut allergies.

Oats, wheat germ, and dried fruit are all rich in **fiber**, which helps with **digestion**, and nuts and seeds are a good source of **protein**. Dried cranberries help to fight bladder, kidney, and urinary-tract infections.

1 Dry-fry the seeds and nuts in a skillet over a medium heat, stirring constantly, until they begin to brown—this only takes a couple of minutes. Transfer to a bowl.

2 Dry-fry the coconut chips or desiccated coconut for a minute until lightly golden. Add to the bowl of seeds and nuts. Add all the other ingredients to the bowl and mix everything together.

3 Serve with your choice of milk, yogurt, or fruit juice and fresh fruit.

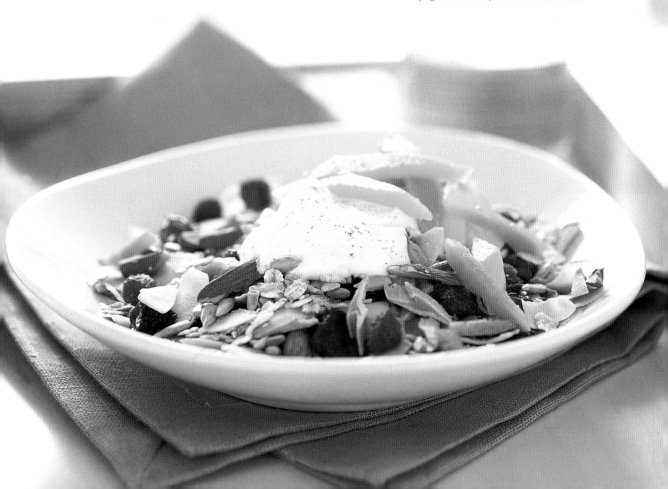

cooked breakfasts

smoked herring with whole-wheat toast

Serves: 2

2 fresh, plump kipper fillets
pat of butter
handful of flat-leaf parsley, roughly chopped
freshly ground black pepper

Whole-wheat toast, to serve

If you have never cooked smoked herrings before, it is worth remembering
that broiling the fish will intensify its flavor and give it a slight crust. Poaching, on the other hand, tends to lessen its flavor but will make it more succulent. Herring are a very good source of **essential fats**, which are important for a developing fetus.

1 Bring a large saucepan of water to a boil. Add the herring, return to a boil, and remove from the heat. Leave for three minutes, drain well.

2 Dot with a little butter and sprinkle with parsley and freshly ground black pepper. Serve immediately with toast.

passion fruit & pineapple muffins

Makes: 12

½ cup less 1 tbsp butter
½ cup soft brown sugar
½ cup vanilla yogurt
2 eggs
8 passion fruit, halved
15-oz can crushed pineapple
zest of ½ lime
juice of 1 lime
3 cups self-rising flour

Anything can be thrown into muffins. But these work particularly well because the pineapple helps to keep them wonderfully moist.

1 Preheat the oven to 350°F. Grease the muffin pans.

2 Puree the butter, sugar, yogurt, and eggs in a food processor until smooth. Add the passion-fruit pulp, pineapple, and lime zest and juice.

3 Fold in the flour, spoon into the muffin pans, and bake for 25–30 minutes.

sweet potato frittata

Serves: 2

1 cup sweet potato, peeled and chopped into small pieces

2 cups spinach

½ cup peas

2 tbsp olive oil

½ onion, peeled and finely chopped

4 eggs

freshly ground black pepper

Sweet potatoes are a very good source of **betacarotene**, which helps to boost the immune system. Spinach is a very good source of **iron** and **folic acid**, and eggs provide **protein**.

1 Bring a saucepan of water to a boil, add the sweet potato, and cook for about 10–15 minutes, until tender. Drain and puree in a food processor or blender.

2 Heat a little water in a saucepan and add the spinach and peas. Cook for one to two minutes, until the spinach has wilted, then drain.

3 Heat half the oil in a small skillet and sauté the onion until soft.

4 In a bowl, whisk the eggs, add the onion, puréed sweet potato, spinach, and peas, and give it a quick stir without totally blending everything together. Season with a little freshly ground black pepper.

5 Heat the rest of the oil in a small skillet, turn the heat down, and pour the egg mixture into the pan. Leave to cook until the egg has almost set (about five minutes). Preheat a broiler to high and finish cooking the frittata under the broiler. Serve in wedges.

lunches

wraps

cream cheese & spinach

Serves: 2

2 flour tortillas
cream cheese
1 handful of cherry tomatoes, halved
2 handfuls of baby spinach leaves, washed and dried
freshly ground black pepper

Tortillas are a source of **fiber**, which helps with digestion. Cream cheese provides **calcium**, which helps strengthen bones. Spinach leaves are a good source of **folic acid**, which helps prevent birth defects in early pregnancy.

1 Spread the flour tortillas with cream cheese. Cover with cherry tomato halves and spinach leaves, and wrap up.

2 If you prefer them warm, wrap in foil and put into a hot oven for five to 10 minutes. Otherwise, eat them as they are.

herby cannellini

Serves: 2–3

⅔ cup canned cannellini beans, drained and rinsed
1 cup mackerel or tuna, drained
½ tsp finely chopped rosemary
a few basil leaves, shredded
1 each small celery stalk, tomato, and shallot, peeled; all finely chopped
handful of baby Little Gem lettuce leaves, finely shredded
2–3 flour tortillas

for the dressing:
2 tbsp red wine vinegar
3 tbsp extra virgin olive oil
1 clove garlic, peeled and minced
sea salt and freshly ground black pepper

This would also be delicious served with warm new potatoes and an arugula and watercress salad. Another good bean idea is to mix together canned red kidney beans, cream cheese, sliced scallions, and freshly chopped cilantro.

Cannellini beans are an excellent source of **protein** and **fiber**, which provide energy and help with digestion. Canned fish is excellent for **calcium**, helping the body with growth and development.

1 Bring a pan of water to a boil, add the beans, and blanch for a few minutes. Drain and transfer to a bowl. Mash the beans slightly.
2 Mix together the dressing ingredients and add to the beans in the bowl with all the remaining ingredients, except the

lettuce and tortillas. Mix thoroughly and season to taste.
3 Scatter the lettuce leaves over the tortillas, cover with the bean spread, and roll up the wraps. Cut in half and serve.

mozzarella, caramelized red onion & arugula

Serves: 3–4

2 tbsp olive oil
3 red onions, peeled and finely sliced
1 tbsp soft brown sugar
2-3 tsp balsamic vinegar
2½ cups wild arugula
5 flour tortillas
1½ cups mozzarella, thinly sliced

Be creative with other fillings; tortillas are great with lots of different flavors. Try meats, cheeses, pestos, and roasted tomatoes. There is a fine line between too much filling and not quite enough—if you are too generous, the wraps don't stay neatly rolled, but skimp and you feel slightly cheated.

Mozzarella is a very good source of **calcium**, which helps to keep bones strong. Wild arugula provides **iron** and **folic acid**, which aid in growth and development.

1 Heat the oil in a skillet, add the onions, and cook gently for 15 minutes, until starting to caramelize. Add the sugar and balsamic vinegar. Cook for another 10 minutes, until the onions are sweet and sticky.

2 Lay the wild arugula on the tortillas, arrange a few slices of mozzarella strips in the middle of the tortillas, and cover with a layer of caramelized onions.

3 Roll up the tortillas and seal in plastic wrap. Refrigerate for at least 30 minutes before serving. Cut each wrap in half and serve.

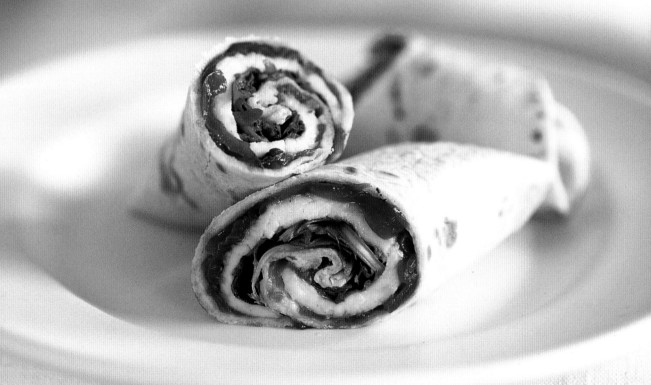

sandwiches

pesto tuna with tomato & watercress

Serves: 2

1⅓ cup tuna canned in oil, drained

2–3 tbsp fresh pesto—to taste, depending on the pesto used

squeeze of lemon juice

freshly ground black pepper

2 chunks of baguette or rolls

2 ripe tomatoes, sliced

handful of watercress leaves

This recipe makes two sandwiches—halve the quantity if you only want one.

Tuna provides **phosphorus**, while baguettes offer **complex carbohydrates**—both help to produce energy. Tomatoes are an excellent source of **vitamin C**, which helps the healing processes in the body.

1 Put the tuna into a bowl, add the pesto, lemon juice, and pepper to taste, and mix together.

2 Spread this mixture onto the chunks of baguette or into the rolls. Cover with the tomato slices and watercress, and the other slices of bread. Wrap up and take to work.

parmesan, pear & arugula with a balsamic dressing

Serves: 1–2

1 ripe pear

2 granary rolls or bread of your choice

handful each of arugula and watercress

handful of Parmesan cheese shavings

for the dressing:

1 tbsp balsamic vinegar

2 tbsp extra-virgin olive oil

a little squeeze of lime juice

freshly ground black pepper

Pear and bread are both sources of **fiber**, which help with the digestive system. Arugula and watercress both provide **vitamin C**, which helps to boost the immune system.

1 Core the pear, cut into slices, and put into the rolls or onto the bread. Add the rocket, watercress, and Parmesan.

2 Mix together the dressing ingredients and drizzle as much or as little as you like into the rolls or onto the bread.

smoked mackerel with horseradish & apple

Serves: 2–3

2–3 smoked mackerel fillets, skinned
2–3 tbsp creamed horseradish
slices of rye or whole-wheat bread
2 apples, cored and sliced
juice of 1 lime
freshly ground black pepper

Oily fish are great sources of **essential fatty acids**, which help with the growth process. Apples and limes are good sources of **vitamin C**, which boosts the immune system.

1 Flake the fish into large pieces, and spread the horseradish onto the slices of rye or whole-wheat bread. Top with the mackerel fillets.

2 Toss the apple slices in a bowl with the lime juice, arrange on top of the fish, and season with pepper.

fennel & pepper

Serves: 2

1 fennel bulb
4 slices sun-dried tomato loaf
2 tbsp black olive or sun-dried tomato paste
3 red peppers, raw or roasted, seeded and thinly sliced

for the dressing:
1 tsp Dijon mustard
juice of ½ lemon
2 tbsp extra virgin olive oil
handful of fresh flat-leaf parsley, finely chopped
sea salt and freshly ground black pepper

Whenever possible, try to pack raw vegetables into your sandwiches. Raw fennel is crisp, juicy, and has a licorice flavor; you will need to keep it very thinly sliced to make sure that the flavor is not too strong.

The sun-dried tomato loaf contains **fiber**, which helps with digestion. Red peppers are a very good source of **vitamin C**, which helps boost the body's immune system.

1 Halve the fennel lengthways, then slice very thinly into strips.
2 Spread the bread with olive or sun-dried tomato paste and top with the sliced peppers.

3 Mix together the dressing ingredients and season well.
4 Spoon over the peppers, cover with the other slices of bread to make sandwiches, and enjoy.

salads

fish salad with herb vinaigrette

Serves: 2

10 cherry tomatoes, halved
sea salt and freshly ground black pepper
1 tbsp extra-virgin olive oil
1 tsp balsamic vinegar
3 large handfuls of arugula
12 oz hot smoked trout fillets
8 cooked large or jumbo shrimp, shelled
2 tbsp capers

for the dressing:
2 tbsp each chopped dill and chives,
sunflower oil, olive oil, and red wine vinegar
1 tsp Dijon mustard
pinch of sugar
freshly ground black pepper

Cherry tomatoes are good for **vitamin C**, a powerful antioxidant. Oil-rich fish, such as trout, provide **essential fats**, which are essential for a developing fetus, and shrimp are a good source of **calcium, magnesium**, and **protein**. Shrimp must be cooked thoroughly.

1 Preheat the oven to 350°F. Put the cherry tomatoes in a roasting pan, season, and drizzle with oil. Roast for 10 minutes in the oven, then drizzle over the balsamic vinegar and roast for another 15 minutes, until lightly wilted. Leave to cool.
2 Make the dressing; put the ingredients into a screw-top jar, replace the lid, and shake well until thick and emulsified.
3 Scatter the arugula over serving plates, top with the smoked trout and shrimp, and scatter over with the capers and tomatoes. Drizzle over with the dressing and serve with hunks of fresh crusty bread.

new potato salad with bacon & avocado

Serves: 3

5 slices of lean or fatty bacon
3½ cups new potatoes
handful of flat-leaf parsley, roughly chopped
2 carrots, washed or peeled and trimmed
2 celery stalks
1 avocado, peeled and stoned
large handful of watercress, roughly chopped
2 red peppers, seeded and finely sliced
sea salt and freshly ground black pepper

for the vinaigrette dressing:
1½ tbsp lemon juice
3 tbsp extra-virgin olive oil
sea salt and freshly ground black pepper

Make this salad and eat for lunch on its own or for supper with a piece of broiled chicken or fish. Potatoes are very good **carbohydrates**, providing energy for the body. Carrots provide **betacarotene**, which is essential for good vision.

1 Preheat a broiler and cook the bacon until crispy.
2 Cook the potatoes in boiling water for about 10–12 minutes, until tender when pierced with a knife. Drain and cut in half.
3 Make the dressing; whisk the lemon juice and oil together and season well. Pour the dressing over the warm potatoes in a salad bowl (they will absorb the flavor from the dressing into their flesh). Add the parsley and mix everything together. Leave to stand for 10 minutes.
4 Thinly slice the carrots, celery, and avocado. Add the watercress and red pepper to the potatoes. Mix everything together, season to taste, and serve.

fennel & roast beet salad

Serves: 4

2 fennel bulbs

4 beets

1 tbsp balsamic vinegar

7 cups mixed watercress, arugula, and spinach

couple of handfuls each of sunflower and pumpkin seeds, toasted

for the dressing:

1 tbsp balsamic

3 tbsp olive oil

1 large clove garlic, finely chopped

½-inch piece of fresh ginger root, peeled and grated

sea salt and freshly ground black pepper

If you want to make this slightly more substantial, serve with cottage cheese and bread.

Beets are a source of **folic acid**, which is very important in helping to prevent birth defects in the early stages of pregnancy. Mixed lettuce leaves provide **betacarotene**, which helps to boost the immune system and the seeds are a great source of **essential fatty acids**.

1 Preheat the oven to 350°F. Slice the fennel into thin wedges. Wrap the beets (with skin on) in foil parcels.

2 Arrange the beets in a roasting pan and roast in the oven for 30 minutes. Add the fennel and roast for another 10 minutes.

3 Drizzle the balsamic vinegar over the fennel and roast for another 10 minutes.

4 Slice the beets into wedges and put into a bowl. Add the fennel and mixed leaves.

5 Mix together the dressing ingredients. Drizzle the dressing over the salad and sprinkle over with the seeds.

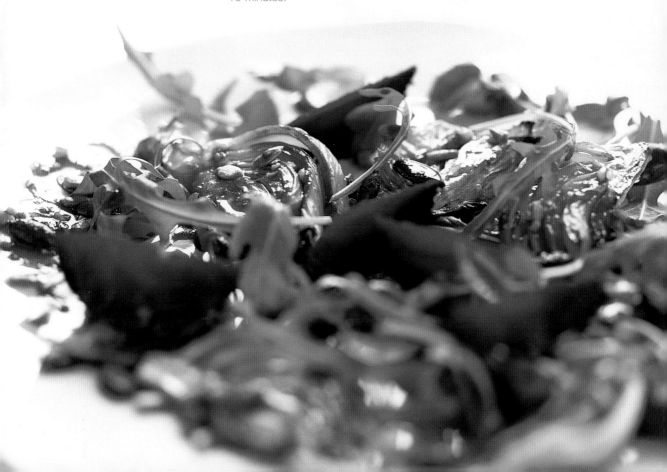

"anything goes" salad with a honey & mint dressing

Serves: 3–4

handful of sunflower seeds

4 cups baby spinach leaves, washed and sorted

handful of cherry tomatoes, quartered

handful of radishes, sliced

2 small beets, peeled and diced

for the dressing (this dressing makes enough for four):

handful of mint, finely chopped

1–2 cloves garlic, crushed

1 tsp liquid honey

½–1 tsp Dijon mustard, to taste

sea salt and freshly ground black pepper

2 tbsp red-wine vinegar

4 tbsp extra-virgin olive oil

a couple of nice cheeses, e.g. Cheddar and Jarlsberg or smoked mackerel fillets, and fresh bread, to serve

Chose your favorite salad ingredients and add to the bowl—as long as you add some spinach. This is great served with smoked mackerel and fresh crusty bread.

There are quite a few benefits from the ingredients in this salad, depending on what you choose to throw in. To give you an idea: sunflower seeds contain **magnesium**, which is involved in producing energy; spinach is great for **iron**, which is essential to the development and growth of an unborn child; tomatoes are a good source of **vitamin C**, which assists in the absorption of iron; and beets are a good source of **folic acid**, which helps to reduce risks of spina bifida in the early stages of pregnancy.

1 Put the sunflower seeds into a dry skillet and heat gently for a few minutes. Transfer to a large bowl and add all of the other salad ingredients.

2 Put the dressing ingredients into a screw-top jar, replace the lid, and shake well to mix. Pour the dressing over the salad, toss everything together, and serve with chunks of hard cheese or mackerel fillets and slices of fresh crusty bread.

romaine lettuce, pear & Parmesan salad

Serves: 3–4

⅔ cup hazelnuts, chopped
2 small pears, peeled and cored
squeeze of lemon juice
2 heads of romaine, washed and torn
1 cup Parmesan cheese shavings

for the dressing:
3 tbsp extra-virgin olive oil
1 tbsp lemon juice
sea salt and freshly ground black pepper

Pears provide **fiber**, which helps with digestion. Hazelnuts are very high in **vitamin E**, which helps maintain healthy skin. Parmesan cheese provides **calcium**, which helps to prevent osteoporosis.

1 Dry-fry the hazelnuts in a skillet, moving them around regularly until golden in color.
2 Slice the pears into chunks and cover in lemon juice to prevent browning. Put into a bowl with the hazelnuts and lettuce.

3 Make the dressing; mix the oil and lemon juice together, and season. Pour the dressing over the salad and finish with fresh Parmesan shavings.

chickpea salad with cumin & yogurt dressing

Serves: 4

½ cucumber
3⅓ cups chickpeas, drained
handful of cherry tomatoes, finely chopped

for the dressing:
1 tsp cumin seeds, dry-fried and ground
2 tbsp plain yogurt
handful of mint leaves, finely sliced
sea salt and freshly ground black pepper

This is quick and easy to make, and tastes fabulous. Cumin has quite a powerful flavor—add more or less to suit your taste.

Chickpeas provide **protein,** and cucumber is a source of **folic acid**, which is essential in the manufacture of **amino acids** and red blood cells.

Tomatoes are a good source of **vitamin C**, which strengthens the body's immune system.

1 Cut the cucumber in half lengthways, scoop out the seeds, and cut the flesh into small pieces or strips.
2 Put the chickpeas into a bowl and add the cucumber and cherry tomatoes.

3 Mix together the dressing ingredients and pour over the salad. Toss everything together and serve.

soups

butternut squash & cumin soup

Serves: 6

1 tbsp olive oil

1 large onion, peeled and finely chopped

2 medium cloves garlic, peeled and minced

½ tsp cumin seeds

½ tsp ground cumin

7 cups butternut squash, peeled & chopped into cubes

4 cups vegetable stock

1 tbsp tomato paste

freshly ground black pepper

a little skim milk (optional)

Butternut squash is very high in **betacarotene**, which is essential for growth and a healthy immune system.

1 Heat the oil in a large saucepan and sauté the onion until soft. Add the garlic, cumin seeds, and ground cumin, and cook for another minute.
2 Mix in the butternut squash, add the stock and tomato paste, and bring to a boil. Cover with a lid and simmer for 30 minutes, until the pumpkin is very soft.
3 Using a hand blender, puree the soup until smooth. Season with black pepper. If the mixture is too thick, thin it with some skim milk.

pea soup

Serves: 6

1 tbsp olive oil, plus extra for drizzling

1 large onion, peeled and finely chopped

1 clove garlic, peeled and sliced

5⅓ cups frozen peas

4 cups vegetable stock

handful of mint leaves

¾ cup Parmesan cheese, freshly grated

Served with Parmesan, mint, and olive oil. This is the perfect soup for when you have no fresh vegetables in the house. Freeze any left over in plastic bags and heat through as and when needed.

Peas provide **protein**, helping the body in growth and development. They also contain **folic acid**, which can help to prevent birth defects.

1 Heat the oil in a large saucepan and sauté the onion and garlic. Add two-thirds of the peas, stock, and the mint, reserving some leaves for scattering. Cover and bring to a boil, then simmer for five minutes.
2 Puree the mixture in a food processor or blender. Return to the pan, add the remaining peas and stock, and simmer for five minutes.
3 Serve in warm soup bowls— spoon the Parmesan into the middle of each, scatter over the remaining mint leaves, and drizzle with olive oil.

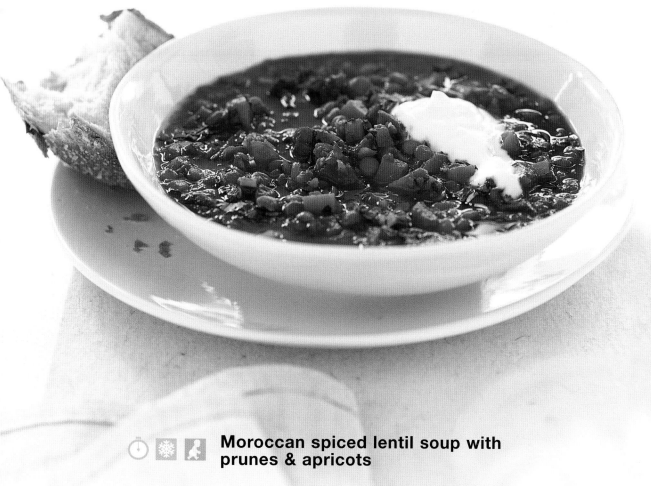

Moroccan spiced lentil soup with prunes & apricots

Serves: 4

2 tbsp olive oil

5 carrots, peeled and chopped

2 celery stalkks, chopped

2 onions, peeled and chopped

5 cloves garlic, peeled and minced

1 tsp each cinnamon, allspice, and cumin

1⅓ cup green lentils

1½ cups chopped canned tomatoes

1 cup fruity red wine

8 cups chicken stock

14 pieces mixed prunes and apricots

handful each of parsley and mint, chopped

Lentils provide protein, which helps with growth and development. Prunes and apricots provide **fiber**, which aids the digestion process.

1 Heat the oil in a large saucepan and sauté the carrots, celery, and onions for about five minutes. Add the garlic and sauté for another five minutes, until the vegetables begin to soften.

2 Add the spices and coat the vegetables, releasing their aroma.

3 Add the lentils, tomatoes, red wine, and stock. Bring to a boil and simmer, uncovered, for about 40 minutes, by which time the lentils should be cooked through.

4 Add the fruit and gently cook for another 10 minutes. Roughly puree in a food processor and stir in the herbs. If you like, serve it with a dollop of plain strained yogurt on top and fresh, crusty bread.

something hot

avocado & pepper tortilla pizzas

A very quick and easy way to eat a few more vegetables.

Flour tortillas make great pizza bases (as long as you like them thin and crispy), and they come in a multitude of flavors—for example, garlic and cilantro. Try other toppings to suit your taste. Anchovies, pesto, mozzarella, tuna, and sweetcorn are all scrumptious.

Red peppers and chilies are an excellent source of **vitamin C**, which is essential for growth and development. Avocados provide **vitamin E,** which helps to maintain healthy skin, and flour tortillas are a source of **carbohydrates**.

Makes: 3 pizzas

1 red pepper, halved and seeded
1 large avocado
2–3 scallions
1 red chili, seeded
3 flour tortillas
6 tbsp tomato paste
handful of cherry tomatoes, sliced
handful of black olives, pitted and sliced
⅔ cup Cheddar cheese, finely grated

1 Thinly slice the red pepper. Cut the avocado in half and remove the seed. Peel and thinly slice the flesh. Thinly slice the scallions and the chili diagonally.

2 Spread each tortilla with one to two tablespoons tomato paste, scatter over with the pepper, avocado, tomatoes, scallions, chili, and olives, and top each with grated cheese.

3 Broil for three to five minutes, until the tortillas are crisp and golden and the cheese has melted.

other topping ideas

Thinly sliced tomatoes, wilted spinach, slices of broiled bacon, and grated Parmesan.

Tuna, anchovies, sliced and sautéed red onion, and lightly blanched broccoli.

Sliced tomatoes, crispy pancetta, grated cheese, olives, and finely chopped chili or a sprinkling of chili powder.

penne with an instant tomato sauce & herbs

Serves: 4

2½ cups penne or other small-sized pasta of your choice

1 cup sun-dried cherry tomatoes in olive oil

1 clove garlic, peeled and roughly chopped

1 shallot, peeled and roughly chopped

sea salt and freshly ground black pepper

2 tsp aged balsamic vinegar (try and find a good one, but don't worry if you can't)

2 tbsp extra virgin olive oil, plus extra for drizzling

6 basil leaves, chopped

bag of arugula leaves, to serve

Serve this pasta dish with a fresh green salad.

Pasta is a great **complex carbohydrate**, which provides slow-release energy to the body. Cherry tomatoes contain **betacarotene** and **vitamin C**, both of which help boost the immune system.

1 Bring a large saucepan of water to a boil. Add the pasta, and cook according to the instructions on the package.

2 Blitz the remaining ingredients, except the basil and arugula, in a food processor for a few seconds, until the mixture resembles a chunky salsa. Mix with the cooked pasta.

3 Drizzle with a little extra olive oil and sprinkle with chopped basil. Serve hot or cold with the arugula or any other green lettuce leaves.

suppers
meat & poultry

chicken, chickpea & sweet potato stew

Serves: 4

1 small organic chicken

5 cloves garlic

4 tbsp extra-virgin olive oil

sea salt and freshly ground black pepper

½ onion,

1 celery stalk

1 bay leaf

a few peppercorns

4 leeks, trimmed and sliced

1 tbsp sage leaves

2 tbsp lemon juice

2 sweet potatoes, peeled and chopped into small pieces

1½ cup canned chickpeas, drained

olive oil, handful of fresh Parmesan cheese shavings, and crusty bread, to serve

This is delicious served in big bowls with chunks of fresh bread for mopping up the juices. If you do not have time to make your own stock, use the best vegetable bouillon powder you can buy. You could always roast a large chicken for supper one night and keep some of the meat to make this stew the next day.

Chicken is a very good source of **protein, minerals,** and **essential B vitamins,** all of which assist with growth and development. Chickpeas are a very good source of **protein** and **soluble fiber,** giving the body energy. Sweet potatoes are an excellent source of **betacarotene,** which strengthens the immune system.

1 Preheat the oven to 350°F. Put the chicken in a roasting pan, add the garlic cloves, drizzle with two tablespoons of the oil, and season well. Roast for 20 minutes a pound plus an extra 10 minutes.

2 Carve the chicken meat, put the chicken carcass (without any skin) into a saucepan. Cover with cold water (approximately four cups), add half an onion and a stalk of celery, a bay leaf and a few peppercorns, and bring to a boil. Simmer for 20 minutes and strain.

3 Heat the remaining oil in a saucepan, add the leeks, and sauté for five minutes. Add the soft roasted garlic, sage, lemon juice, chicken stock, sweet potato, and chickpeas, simmer for 10 minutes, add enough chicken for four, and cook for another five minutes or until all of the vegetables are cooked.

4 Serve with olive oil and Parmesan shavings on top and crusty bread for dipping.

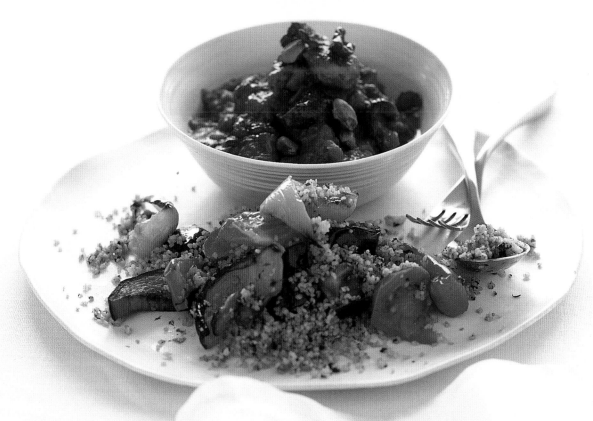

Moroccan lamb with saffron and apricots

Serves: 6

Serve with the Spicy Couscous with Roasted Vegetables, page 120, or with rice.

Lamb provides **protein** and **iron**, which are essential for a developing fetus. Tomatoes are a good source of **betacarotene** and **vitamin C**, which help boost the immune system.

large pinch of saffron threads (about 20)

4 tbsp olive oil

3¼ lb lamb for stew, cut into bite-size pieces

2 cups pearl onions, peeled

3 cloves garlic, peeled and finely minced

2 tbsp grated fresh ginger root

1½ tbsp ground coriander

2 tsp ground cumin, plus extra, to taste

large pinch of cayenne pepper

½ tsp cinnamon and 1 cinnamon stick

3 tsp harissa paste, plus extra, to taste

1¾ cups crushed tomatoes

4 cups chicken stock

⅓ cup each apricots, dates, and prunes

sea salt and freshly ground black pepper

2 tbsp butter

⅓ cup each almonds, pistachios, and dried cranberries

1 Mix the saffron with one tablespoon of boiling water and let stand. Heat half the oil in a large skillet and cook the lamb in batches for two to three minutes. Transfer to an ovenproof dish and keep warm.

2 Pour off all but one tablespoon of the oil from the pan, lower the heat, and cook the onions for five minutes, until golden. Stir in the saffron, garlic, ginger, spices, and harissa, and cook for one minute.

3 Add the tomatoes, stock, and fruit, bring to the boil, and season well. Stir in the lamb, cover and simmer, stirring occasionally, for 1½ hours, or until tender. Add the ground cumin and harissa to taste.

4 Heat the butter in a small saucepan, add the nuts and cranberries, and sauté for a couple of minutes. Spoon the lamb into a warm serving dish and scatter with the buttery nuts and fruit.

sautéed chicken breast with a mustard sauce

Serves: 4

1 tbsp butter
1 tbsp olive oil
4 chicken breasts
2 shallots, peeled and finely chopped
⅓ cup white wine
1 cup chicken stock
2 cloves garlic, finely minced
⅔ cup whipping cream
1 tbsp whole-grain mustard
1 tbsp chopped tarragon
2 tsp finely chopped thyme
1 tbsp chopped parsley for scattering
sea salt and freshly ground black pepper

boiled potatoes or rice and
wilted spinach, to serve

The beauty of this dish is that it takes very little time to throw together and you can start to prepare it a little while before you need and then finish it off before serving.

Chicken is a good source of **protein**, which helps with growth and development. Whipping cream provides some **calcium**, helping to strengthen teeth and bones.

1 Heat the butter and the oil in a heavy skillet over a medium-high heat. Add the chicken breasts and sauté for a few minutes on each side, until golden brown—this seals in the juices. Using a slotted spoon, transfer to a dish and keep warm.

2 Heat any oil and butter left in the skillet, then add the shallots and sauté for one minute, until softened.

3 Add the wine, stock, and garlic, and bring to a boil. Boil until the liquid has reduced to about ½ cup.

4 Whisk in the cream and mustard and bring back to a boil. Cook until slightly thickened. Add the thyme, season to taste, and whisk thoroughly.

5 Return the chicken breasts to the skillet and cook for five minutes, until cooked through but not overcooked. Scatter with fresh parsley and serve with potatoes or rice and wilted spinach.

Chinese-style honey-glazed duck with sweet & sticky pak choi

Serves: 4

4 duck breasts
1 tbsp Chinese five-spice powder
1 tbsp and 1 tsp liquid honey
2 tsp soy sauce
5 cups bok choy, shredded
1 tbsp olive oil
1 red chili, seeded and finely chopped
2 cloves garlic, peeled and finely minced
1 tbsp finely chopped fresh ginger root
1 tbsp hoisin
1 tbsp mirin

Pak choi can be green- or white-stemmed and it comes in many shapes and sizes. Mirin is a form of sweetened sake, which is available from good supermarkets.

Chicken is a very good source of **protein** and **minerals**, which are vital for growth and development. Pak choi is a good source of **betacarotene** and **vitamin C**, which both strengthen the immune system. Ginger root is thought to relieve morning sickness.

1 Preheat the oven to 400°F. Heat a heavy skillet, add the duck breasts and sear, skin-side down, for a few minutes until brown—you do not need to add any extra oil to the skillet.

2 Mix together the five-spice powder, one tablespoon of the honey, and one tablespoon of the soy sauce, and brush liberally all over the duck breasts. Put onto a baking sheet and roast in the oven for eight minutes—the meat should still be slightly springy to the touch. Leave to rest.

3 Bring a little water to a boil in a saucepan, add the pak choi, and cook for few minutes, until wilted but still slightly crisp in texture.

4 Heat the oil in a skillet, add the chili, garlic, and ginger root, and sauté for a couple of minutes. Add the hoisin, mirin, and the remaining soy sauce and honey. Cook for one minute, then drizzle over the bok choy. Slice the duck and serve with the pak choi.

fish

plaice with a Sicilian stuffing

Serves: 4

4 large plaice fillets, skinned and halved

1–2 tbsp olive oil

for the filling:

2 tbsp each fresh white breadcrumbs and extra virgin olive oil

1 tbsp shredded basil leaves

2 tsp each finely chopped mint and chopped capers

1 tbsp each pine nuts, raisins, and chopped olives

Serve with roasted red peppers, spinach, and a balsamic vinaigrette. Fish and nuts are good sources of protein, which helps with the baby's growth and development. The nuts provide a good source of fat.

1 Preheat the oven to 400°F. Mix all the filling ingredients together. Spoon a teaspoon of the filling on top of each fillet half at the wider end, and roll up.

2 Pack tightly into an ovenproof dish, scatter over any extra stuffing, and drizzle with oil. Bake in the oven for about eight minutes, depending on the size of the fish, until cooked through.

oven-baked lemon & herb risotto with monkfish rosemary skewers

Serves: 4

2 tbsp butter

2 tbsp olive oil

1 onion or 3 shallots, finely chopped

1 cup arborio rice

½ cup white wine

3 cups light vegetable stock

zest of 1 lemon

1¼ lb monkfish tail, cubed

rosemary sprigs for skewering

2 tbsp extra-virgin olive oil

½ cup Parmesan cheese, grated

4 tbsp chopped basil

sea salt and freshly ground black pepper

1 lemon, cut into chunks, to serve

A much less time-consuming way of preparing risotto is to throw it into the oven rather than standing over the stove stirring. There is only a small amount of wine added and the alcohol content is minimal.

1 Preheat the oven to 350°F.
2 Melt the butter and oil in a heavy skillet and sauté the onion or shallots slowly, without coloring, for five to 10 minutes, until softened. Turn the heat up slightly, add the rice to the pan and stir, thoroughly coating with the buttery onion. Stir for a minute or two to coat the grains.
3 Add the wine and let that bubble. Add the stock and bring up to simmering point. Stir once and transfer to a warm ovenproof dish. Put in the middle of the oven, uncovered. After 20 minutes,

remove from the oven, stir once, and add the lemon zest. Return to the oven for 15 minutes.
4 Carefully skewer the fish onto the rosemary and brush with oil. Cover the ends of the rosemary with foil to prevent burning. Cook under a hot broiler for two to three minutes on each side, until cooked through.
5 When the risotto is ready, stir in the Parmesan and basil. Season well and leave to stand for a couple of minutes before serving with the fish and chunks of lemon.

Goan fish curry with chickpea, lemon & spinach rice

Serves: 4

for the rice:

1¼ cup basmati rice

zest of 1 lemon

1½ cups canned chickpeas, drained and rinsed

6½ cups baby spinach

sea salt and freshly ground black pepper

for the fish curry:

2 tbsp vegetable oil

2 onions, peeled and chopped

large piece of fresh ginger root, peeled and chopped

3 cloves garlic, peeled and chopped

2 stalks lemon grass, crushed with a rolling pin

2 red chilies, seeded and finely chopped

3 tsp turmeric

6 cardamom pods

2 tsp garam masala

2–3 tsp medium curry powder

1 lb mixed fresh fish, e.g. monkfish, salmon, and raw jumbo shrimp

½ cup creamed coconut, cut into pieces

Fish and rice are both good sources of **protein**, which is essential for a developing fetus. Creamed coconut provides some **calcium**, which helps to strengthen teeth and bones, and ginger root is thought to be good for relieving morning sickness. Spinach is a good source of **folic acid**, which helps to reduce birth defects during early pregnancy.

1 Put the rice, lemon zest, and 2½ cups water in a saucepan, cover, and bring to a boil.

2 Reduce the heat and simmer, still covered, for exactly 14 minutes. Remove from the heat and quickly add the chickpeas. Cover and leave to stand for exactly nine minutes. Remove the lid and add the spinach. Cover and let stand for another couple of minutes.

3 Make the curry: heat the oil in a saucepan, add the onion, ginger root, garlic, lemon grass, and chilies, and cook for 10 minutes.

Stir constantly without letting the onions brown. Add the turmeric, cardamom pods, garam masala, and curry powder. Mix well and cook for another five minutes.

4 Cut the fish into large chunks, add to spice mix along with ⅛ cup water, and simmer for five minutes. Add the shrimp and cook for another five minutes.

5 Add the creamed coconut and stir carefully until it has melted—it should not boil. Serve with the chickpea and spinach rice.

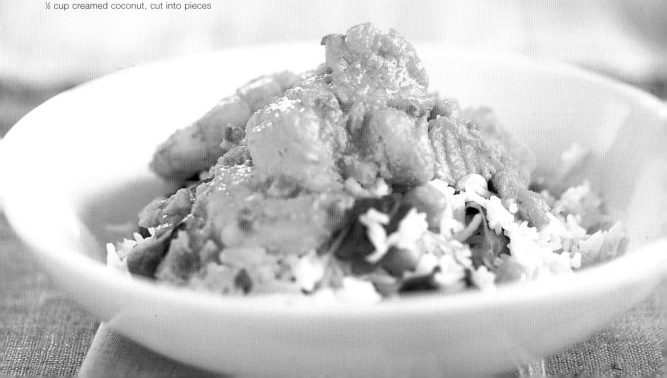

fennel & citrus fruit salmon

Serves: 4

4½ cups new potatoes, scrubbed and cut into small pieces

1 tbsp fennel seeds, roasted and crushed

zest of 1 lime and 1 lemon

1 cup fresh breadcrumbs

4 salmon fillets

sea salt and freshly ground black pepper

1–2 tbsp olive oil

1–2 tsp Dijon mustard

3 cups sugar snap peas

1 lemon, cut into wedges, to serve

The salmon has a subtle but delicious crunchy topping. Serve with potatoes and green vegetables.

Potatoes provide **carbohydrate**, for slow-releasing energy. Salmon is a good source of **protein** and **essential fatty acids**, which are vital for growth and development. Sugar snaps are a good source of **vitamin C**, strengthening the immune system.

1 Preheat the oven to 400°F. Bring a saucepan of water to a boil, add the potatoes, and cook until tender. Mix together the fennel seeds, lime and lemon zests, and breadcrumbs.

2 Season the salmon fillets with salt and pepper. Heat the oil in a heavy ovenproof skillet and sauté the salmon (skin side up) for 30–40 seconds, moving constantly so that they do not stick. Turn over and sauté for another 30 seconds, moving around in the skillet. Remove from the heat, brush the salmon with the mustard, and sprinkle over a layer of the crumb mixture, packing it onto the salmon. Place the skillet on the top shelf of the oven and cook for four to five minutes until cooked through.

3 Meanwhile, blanch the sugar snap peas in boiling water for a minute. Remove the fish from the oven and let rest for a few minutes before serving with lemon wedges, the boiled potatoes, and sugar snap peas.

spiced lentils with shrimp

(prepare lentils ahead)

Serves: 4

2 cup Puy lentils

1½ cups water

2 scallions, finely sliced

2 tbsp extra virgin olive oil

2 tbsp red wine vinegar

1 red chili, seeded, finely chopped

sea salt and freshly ground black pepper

1 tsp each ground coriander, ground cumin, and turmeric

½ cup cilantro leaves, chopped

20 raw shrimps, shelled

1 cupgreen beans

5 cups baby spinach leaves

handful of mint leaves

for the dressing:

⅓ cup plain yogurt

2 tbsp lime juice

4 tbsp chopped mint

This is incredibly tasty, low in fat, and packed with nutrients.

Lentils and shrimp are a good source of **protein**, which is important for growth and development. Shrimp must be cooked thoroughly.

1 Place the lentils and water in a medium saucepan and bring to a boil. Reduce the heat and simmer for 15 minutes. Drain the lentils.

2 Put the warm lentils, scallions, one tablespoon of the olive oil, vinegar, chili, salt and pepper, ground coriander, cumin, ½ tsp of the turmeric, and half the fresh cilantro in a bowl, stir to combine, and set aside.

3 Put the remaining oil, turmeric, fresh cilantro, and seasoning in a bowl and stir to combine. Add the shrimp and stir to coat.

4 Heat a nonstick skillet, add the shrimp, and cook for a couple of minutes, until they turn pink all over, shaking the skillet frequently.

5 Bring a little water in a saucepan to a boil, add the green beans, and blanch for a couple of minutes, then add the spinach and let it wilt for a minute.

6 To serve, divide the lentils among four plates, top with the beans, spinach, mint, and shrimp. Mix together the dressing ingredients and drizzle over the salad.

vegetarian

spicy couscous with roasted vegetables

Serves: 6

2 each red and yellow peppers, seeded

2 medium eggplant

8 ripe tomatoes, halved

6 cloves garlic, peeled

2 red onions, peeled and sliced into thin wedges

2 tbsp olive oil

sea salt and freshly ground black pepper

2¾ cups couscous

3¼ cups boiling vegetable stock (or enough to cover couscous)

large pat butter

1 tsp crushed dried red chili

2–3 tsp harissa paste

for the chermoula:

1 tsp each fennel and cumin seeds, toasted and ground

3 cups cilantro, roughly chopped

½ cup mint, roughly choppped

2 cups parsley, roughly chopped

3 tsp paprika

large pinch of cayenne

pinch of salt

3 cloves garlic, peeled and roughly chopped

zest of 1 orange

1 cup olive oil

The chermoula gives the couscous a wonderful flavor. However, if you are short of time, omit the chermoula and serve the couscous with roasted vegetables—it is still a great dish.

Couscous is a **complex carbohydrate,** providing energy to the body. Peppers, tomatoes, and eggplant are all sources of **vitamin C,** which provides natural immunity.

1 Preheat the oven to 400°F. Cut the peppers into chunks and slice the eggplant. Arrange all the vegetables in a roasting pan, pour over the oil, and toss around until coated. Season, and roast in the oven for 35–45 minutes, turning once, until cooked and golden at the edges.

2 Put the couscous into an ovenproof dish, cover the grains with boiling stock, and leave for 10 minutes for the grains to swell. Dot the butter over the top, season, and sprinkle with the chili. Cover with foil and bake alongside the vegetables for 25 minutes.

3 Meanwhile, make the chermoula: put all the ingredients into a food processor and whiz until smooth. Add the harissa, roasted vegetables, and three to four tablespoons of the chermoula to the couscous. Mix everything together and serve.

NB: serve any leftover chermoula with broiled fish for a quick supper.

squash & thyme tarts with relish

Serves: 6

This makes a perfect supper served with a fresh watercress salad.

for the filling:
14-oz squash, halved and deseeded
1 tbsp olive oil and 2 tbsp butter
1 small leek, trimmed and chopped
2 cloves garlic
1 egg
½ cup Parmesan cheese, grated
⅓ cup heavy cream
¼ cup milk
fresh thyme plus extra sprigs for serving

for the pastry:
1½ cups all-purpose flour
pinch of salt
1 tsp finely chopped thyme
⅓ cup unsalted butter, cut into small pieces and chilled
1 egg
ice-cold water

for the beet and red onion relish:
2 chopped red onions, caramelized
1 cooked beet, finely chopped
1 tbsp balsamic vinegar

1 Preheat the oven to 400°F. Roast the squash for 40 minutes, until soft.

2 Make the pastry: sift the flour and salt into a food processor, add the thyme, and pulse for a few seconds. Add the butter and process to make fine breadcrumbs. Keeping the machine running, add the egg and a little water if necessary, 1 tbsp at a time. If the pastry is still in crumbly pieces, add a little more water. To make by hand, sift the flour into a large bowl with the salt. Add the chopped butter and rub the fat into the flour. Stir in the thyme. Add water a little at a time and bring together to form a ball. Seal in plastic wrap and chill for at least 30 minutes.

3 Roll out the pastry and line four 4-inch tart pans. Chill for 30 minutes.

4 Lower the oven to 350°F. Heat a baking sheet until hot. Cover the pastry with sheets of baking paper and baking beans, place the pans on the tray, and bake for 10 minutes. Remove the paper and beans, and cook for another five minutes.

5 Heat the oil and butter in a small saucepan, add the leek and garlic, and sauté for a few minutes, until soft. Scoop out the cooked squash flesh and put in a food processor with the egg, ¾ of the cheese, cream, milk, and thyme. Process until smooth (or mix well by hand).

6 Fill the tart cases with the squash mixture, top with the remaining cheese. Bake for about 20 minutes, until slightly puffed and golden. Mix together the ingredients for the beet and red onion relish and serve with the tarts.

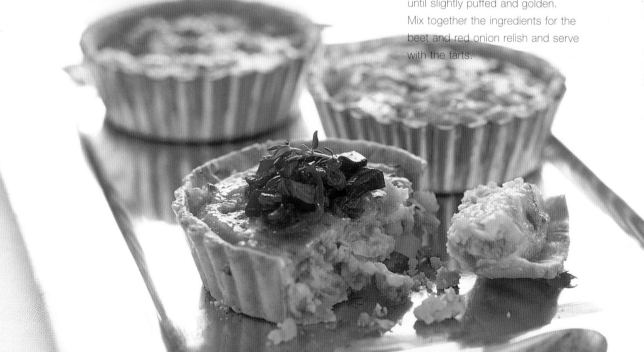

Thai-style curry with tofu

Serves: 4

2 tbsp sesame oil

2 red onions, finely sliced

3 cloves garlic, peeled and finely chopped

2 red chilies, seeded and finely sliced (with a few seeds for a little kick), plus a little chili powder

1½-inch piece of fresh ginger root, peeled and finely chopped

2 tbsp tomato paste

1 stalk lemon grass, crushed with a rolling pin

lime leaves or zest of 1 lime

1⅔ cups soft tofu, cut into small pieces

2 cups sugar snap peas, sliced

1¼ cups coconut milk

1 cup vegetable stock

2–3 tsp fish sauce

3–4 large handfuls of baby spinach leaves

large handful each of cilantro leaves and cashew nuts, chopped and toasted, or sesame seeds or pumpkin seeds, toasted

Tofu is the Japanese name given to soybean curd and is a very good vegetarian source of **protein**, **calcium**, and **iron**, which is essential for a developing fetus. It has the added advantage of being low in saturated fat, contains no cholesterol, and has almost no sodium. Spinach is a good source of **folic acid**, **betacarotene**, and **iron**. Coconut milk also provides some **calcium**, aiding in the development of strong teeth and bones. Ginger root is thought to be very good for relieving morning sickness.

1 Heat the oil in a skillet or wok. Add the onions and fry, stirring well, until deeply colored. Add the garlic, chilies, and ginger, and sauté for another minute, stirring all the time.

2 Add the tomato paste, lemon grass, lime leaves or lime zest, tofu, and sugar snap peas, and stir gently over a medium heat for a minute, to coat the tofu.

3 Add the coconut milk, stock, and fish sauce, and simmer, uncovered, for four minutes. Add the spinach and toss together. Cook for another two minutes. Serve with lots of fresh cilantro, and cashew nuts or seeds scattered over the top.

orange peppers with a brioche filling

Serves: 4

2 orange peppers

2 yellow peppers

1½ cups brioche crumbs
(about 3–4 thick slices)

2 tbsp pine nuts, toasted and
roughly chopped

handful each of flat-leaf parsley and mint

½ lb haloumi cheese

handful of black olives, pitted (optional)

zest of 1 orange

2 tbsp extra virgin olive oil

sea salt and freshly ground black pepper

Brioche is a fabulous sweet, rich bread which makes wonderful crumbs ideal for stuffing roasted peppers.

Haloumi cheese is a very good source of **protein** and **calcium**, which are important for growth and development of strong teeth and bones. Peppers are an excellent source of **vitamin C**, which boosts the immune system. Pine nuts are a very good source of **magnesium** and **zinc**, which are both important for growth.

1 Preheat the oven to 375°F. Put the whole peppers in a roasting pan and roast for 45 minutes, until soft.
2 Put the brioche crumbs onto a baking sheet and toast in the oven for five minutes, turning the crumbs now and then until golden and crisp. Put into a bowl. Add the pine nuts, herbs, cheese, olives, zest, and half the oil to the crumbs, mix together, and season to taste.
3 Remove the stalks from the peppers and scoop out the seeds. Fill the peppers with the crumb mixture and drizzle over the remaining oil. Bake for 15 minutes, until warmed through.

desserts

coconut & cardamom rice pudding

Serves: 4

3 cardamom pods
1 cup pudding rice
1 cup whole or skim milk
1 cup coconut milk
⅓ cup water
few drops of vanilla extract
2 tbsp sugar

The rice is a good source of **carbohydrates**, providing slow-release energy. It is therefore a great dessert to eat at lunchtime.

1 Split the cardamom pods in half, put the seeds into a mortar, and crush with a pestle.
2 Put the rice, milk, coconut milk, water, vanilla, and crushed cardamom seeds into a saucepan. Bring to a boil, then reduce the heat and simmer for about 15–20 minutes, stirring frequently to prevent it from sticking to the bottom. If necessary, add a few tablespoons of water to loosen the mixture.
3 Add the sugar, mix well, and cook for a minute. Serve on its own or with fresh fruit.

little cherry & almond puddings

Makes: 4

for the caramel:
⅓ cup butter
¼ cup sugar
1 tbsp water
1 ½ cup cherries, pitted, plus extra for serving

for the sponge:
½ cup less 1 tbsp softened butter
½ cup sugar
⅓ cup all-purpose flour
½ cup ground almonds
1 tsp baking powder

thick strained plain yogurt, to serve

Serve the puddings with some fresh cherries alongside. Cherries are a great source of **magnesium** and **potassium**.

1 Preheat the oven to 375°F.
2 Make the caramel; melt the butter, sugar, and water together and leave to bubble until golden brown.
3 Butter four small pudding molds or ramekins and divide the pitted cherries among them. Pour over with the caramel.
4 Make the sponge; beat together the butter and sugar. Gradually add the flour, ground almonds, and baking powder. Quickly beat again to mix. Spoon this batter over the cherries.
5 Put the molds onto a tray and bake in the oven for about 30 minutes, until golden and springy to the touch. Let stand for a few minutes, run a knife around the edge of the molds or ramekins, and unmold onto a plate. Serve with a dollop of thick plain strained yoghurt and some extra cherries.

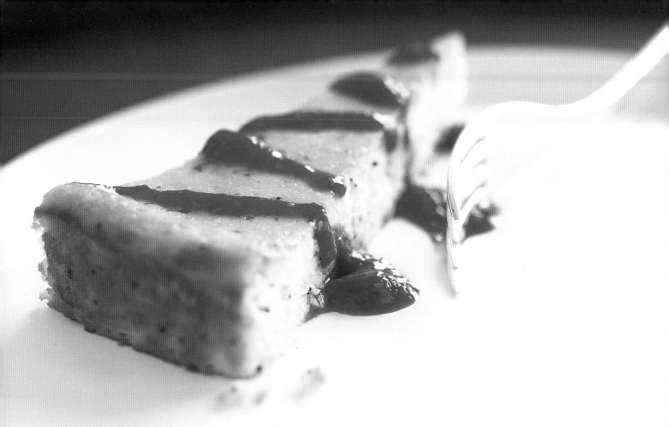

lemon & poppy seed slice with crushed berry sauce

Serves: 6–8

1 cup each cottage cheese and cream cheese
⅔ cup sour cream
¾ cup sugar
juice of 1 lemon
grated zest of 2 lemons
2 tbsp cornstarch
3 organic eggs
1 tbsp poppy seeds

for the sauce:
1⅔ cup raspberries
¼ cup sugar
juice of ½ lemon

The cheeses are great a source of **calcium,** and the fresh raspberries also provide **calcium**, along with **potassium, iron,** and **magnesium**. Raspberries retain their flavor better if they are unwashed, so it is best to choose organic.

1 Preheat the oven to 300°F. Butter and line a 9-in springform flan pan.
2 Put the cheeses, sour cream, sugar, lemon juice and zest, and cornstarch into a food processor and whiz until smooth. Whiz in the eggs one at a time, then stir in the poppy seeds.
3 Pour the mixture into the prepared pan and bake in the oven for about one hour, until just set and slightly puffed. Run a knife around the edge to prevent it from splitting as it cools.
4 Put the ingredients for the raspberry sauce into a food processor and whiz together. Serve in slices with the sauce drizzled over the top.

snacks

things on bruschetta

bruschetta

Take a part-baked ciabatta loaf and bake according to the package instructions. Slice thickly and arrange on a baking sheet. Drizzle with oil and return to the hot oven for a few minutes until crisp and golden. Turn over and cook for a few minutes on the other side. Rub each side with garlic. Munch on these with one of the following toppings.

sardines with lemon & pepper

2 ripe tomatoes, sliced

1 cup sardines in olive oil, drained and oil reserved

freshly ground black pepper

squeeze of lemon

Sardines contain **essential fatty acids**, which are very important for healthy eyes and brain function, especially in unborn babies. Bread is a good source of **fiber**, which helps with digestion. Tomatoes are very rich in **vitamin C**, which is essential for growth.

1 Lay the tomato slices on top of the toasted ciabatta. Arrange the sardines close to each other on the tomatoes, breaking them up slightly with the back of a fork.

Season with pepper and lemon juice. **2** Drizzle with a little olive oil from the sardine can, put under a hot broiler for a minute, and serve.

smashed cannellini beans with lemon

⅔ cup canned cannellini beans, drained and rinsed

1 clove garlic, peeled and crushed

zest and juice of ½–1 lemon

2–3 tbsp extra virgin olive oil, 6 basil leaves

2 tbsp freshly grated Parmesan cheese

Beans are a great source of **fiber** and **protein**.

1 Mash all the ingredients, except the Parmesan, in a bowl, or puree in a food processor or blender.

2 Season with sea salt and black pepper and spread onto the toasted ciabatta. Top with Parmesan to serve.

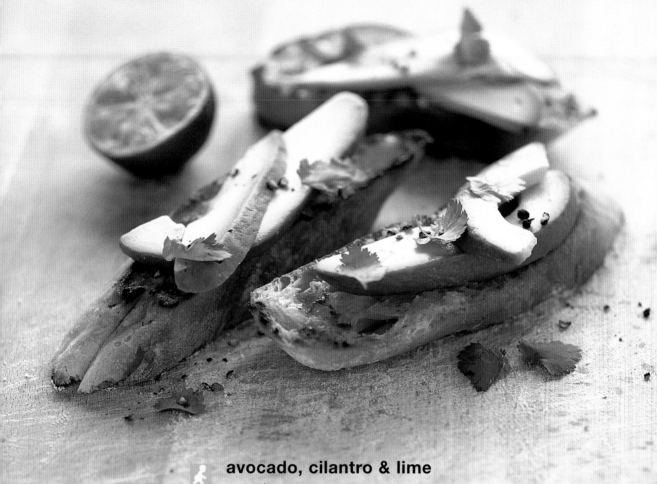

avocado, cilantro & lime

1 avocado
handful of cilantro leaves
juice of ½ lime

Avocados are a good source of **potassium** and **vitamins E** and **A**.

1 Cut the avocado in half and remove the seed. Peel and slice the flesh into strips.

2 Arrange the avocado strips on the ciabatta, scatter over the cilantro, and drizzle with lime juice.

artichoke, lemon & Parmesan

jar of artichokes hearts in oil, drained
squeeze of lemon juice
freshly ground black pepper
2 tbsp finely grated Parmesan cheese
dark-green lettuce leaves

Artichokes supply both **phosphorus** and **iron**, and are also good for the digestion.

1 Lightly mash the artichokes, add the lemon juice and pepper, and spoon onto the ciabatta.

2 Top with the Parmesan. Eat with a handful of fresh green lettuce leaves.

super quick snacks

carrot hummus

1½ cups canned chickpeas, drained and rinsed

3 medium carrots, peeled and chopped

2 tbsp tahini (roasted sesame seed paste)

juice of ½–1 lime or lemon

¼ cup water

3 tbsp olive oil

2 cloves garlic, peeled and crushed

sea salt and freshly ground black pepper

a selection of vegetables, e.g. baby carrots, celery, baby tomatoes, and radishes, and pitta chips, to serve

This will last for a few days in the fridge.

1 Put all the ingredients into a food processor and puree until smooth. Adjust the seasoning to taste.
2 Make the pitta chips; cut the pitta bread in half lengthways, then cut each half into little triangles and toast under a medium broiler for a few minutes, until golden and crisp.
3 Serve the hummus with crudités and/or pitta chips.

roasted pumpkin seeds

bag of pumpkin seeds

2 tsps paprika

good drizzle of olive oil

sea salt and freshly ground black pepper

Pumpkin are particularly favored for their high **zinc**, **calcium**, **B vitamins**, and **essential fatty acid** levels. Eaten regularly, pumpkin seeds can rid the intestinal tract of unwanted parasites.

1 Preheat the oven to 375°F. Spread the pumpkin seeds on a baking sheet and sprinkle with the paprika.
2 Drizzle with oil, season well, and roast in the oven for 10 minutes, turning occasionally. Leave to cool, then store in an airtight container.

nuts & bolts

1 tsp of each cumin seeds, coriander seeds, paprika & black pepper

1¾ cup crunchy cereal of your choice, e.g. toasted granola

1 tbsp each cashews, hazelnuts, pumpkin seeds, sunflower seeds

1 tbsp each dried cranberries, dried, chopped apricots

1-2 tbsp olive oil for drizzling

This is a fun, crunchy snack to munch on. Use any cereal that you like and add spices of your choice, such as Chinese five spice.

1 Preheat the oven to 350°F. Heat the spices in a dry skillet to toast lightly. Crush with a mortar and pestle.

2 Spread the cereal, spices, nuts, and fruit onto a baking sheet. Drizzle with the oil and toss well to coat.

3 Roast in the oven for 15–20 minutes, turning frequently. Leave to cool, store in an airtight container.

fresh ginger tea

Serves: 4–5

4 cups water

3 cardamom pods

1 cinnamon stick

2-inch piece of fresh ginger root, peeled and freshly grated

ice cubes and fresh fruit, e.g. apple and orange slices, to serve (optional)

Try this tea if you are suffering from morning sickness—it may help to relieve some of the symptoms. If you are serving the tea cold, you could always add a few pieces of freshly sliced fruit.

1 Put the water in a saucepan and add the remaining ingredients. Bring to a boil and leave to simmer for three minutes to allow the spices to infuse.

2 Strain the tea and serve hot or chilled with ice cubes and slices of fresh fruit.

breads & cakes

(toddler-friendly if child is tolerant of seeds)·

Makes: one 2-lb loaf

2 eggs

¾ cup milk

½ cup plain yogurt

few drops vanilla extract

2¼ cups all-purpose flour

2 tsp each baking powder and ground cinnamon

1 cup sugar

1¼ cup desiccated coconut

⅔ cup mixed dried fruit, e.g cranberries, cherries, apricots, and pineapple, chopped

¼ cup sunflower seeds, plus extra for sprinkling

¼ cup butter, melted

coconut and fruit bread

Coconut, milk, and plain yogurt all contain **calcium**, which helps to strengthen bones and teeth. Dried fruit is a very good source of **fiber**, which helps with digestion.

1 Preheat the oven to 350°F. Grease and lightly flour a 2-lb loaf pan. Gently whisk together the eggs, milk, yogurt, and vanilla.

2 Sift the flour, baking powder, and cinnamon into a bowl, add the sugar, coconut, fruit, and sunflower seeds, and stir to combine. Make a well in the center and gradually stir in the egg mixture until just combined. Add the melted butter and stir until just smooth, being careful not to overmix.

3 Pour into the prepared pan, sprinkle with sunflower seeds, and bake for 50 minutes to one hour, until a skewer inserted comes out clean. Leave in the pan for five minutes, then transfer to a wire rack and leave to cool.

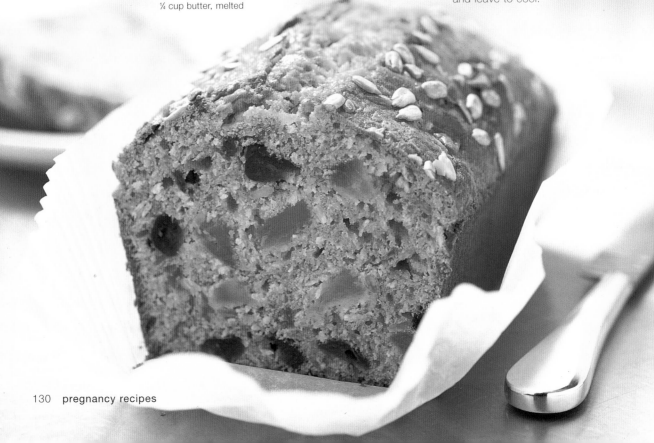

banana, fig, and honey cake

Makes: one 8-inch cake

3 medium eggs

1 cup soft brown sugar

1 cup sunflower oil

⅔ cup milk

1 cup all-purpose flour

1 cup whole-wheat flour

½ tsp bicarbonate soda

1 tsp ground cinnamon

large pinch of nutmeg

1 tsp ground apple or pumpkin pie spice

2 bananas, peeled and mashed

1½ cup dried figs or dates, pitted and chopped

3 tbsps liquid honey

This cake is very easy to make and will keep in an airtight container; alternatively, cut in pieces and put in the freezer. If you feel the urge for a piece of sinful cream-filled cake, eat a piece of this instead.

Bananas are an excellent source of **potassium** and **fiber**, which help with the normal functioning of cells and digestion. They are also very good for energy. Figs, dates, and whole-wheat flour all provide **fiber**, which helps with the digestion process.

1 Preheat the oven to 375°F. Butter and flour an 8-inch cake pan.
2 Put everything into a bowl, except the bananas, figs or dates, and honey, and whisk until mixed together. Stir in the mashed bananas and chopped figs or dates.
3 Spoon into the prepared pan and bake in the oven for 45 minutes to one hour, until a skewer inserted comes out clean. Make holes over the cake with a fork and pour over the honey.

fruity nutty bread

Makes: one 2-lb loaf

2 tbsp sunflower oil

3 cups all-purpose flour

1¼ cups whole-wheat flour

1 tsp sea salt

1 tsp cream of tartar

1 tsp baking soda

1 tsp baking powder

⅔ cup each mixed nuts, toasted and roughly chopped, sunflower seeds, plus extra for sprinkling, and dried apricots, roughly chopped

1 cup plain yogurt

2 tbsp milk

honey

This is a very quick "yeast-free" bread. It is delicious cut into slices and served with a really fruity jam or mashed banana and cinnamon.

1 Preheat the oven to 350°F. Grease a 2-lb loaf pan with half the oil. Sieve the flours, salt, cream of tartar, baking soda, and baking powder together in a large bowl. Stir in the nuts, sunflower seeds, and apricots.
2 Mix together the yogurt, milk, honey, and remaining oil. Stir this yogurt mixture into the dry ingredients and mix to form a soft dough. Spoon the batter into the oiled tin. Sprinkle sunflower seeds over the top.
3 Bake in the oven for one hour—you may need to cover the loaf with waxed paper after 40 minutes to prevent it from going too brown.

breastfeeding
diet

breast
feeding care

Put simply, breast milk provides all the essential nutrients a baby needs for best possible development. There is no substitute.

advantages

Some mothers decide that they don't want to try breastfeeding, and instead bottle-feed their babies from birth.

When you look at the list of advantages to both the baby and the mother, you can see why it is so important.

Put simply, breast milk provides all the essential nutrients a baby needs for the best possible development. There is no substitute.

Of course, some mothers do have problems with breastfeeding, but for those who are able to make the choice, breast is certainly best.

The British Department of Health recommends that "mothers should be encouraged and supported in breastfeeding for at least four months and may choose to continue to breastfeed as the weaning diet becomes increasingly varied."

breastfeeding benefits

- You can usually begin to breastfeed your baby within an hour after birth. The first milk that a mother produces is called colostrum —a yellowish transparent fluid— which is usually excreted for the first three days. It contains less fat, more protein, and more protective factors than the breast milk that is produced later on. These protective factors can help fight polio, mumps, and E. coli.

- Colostrum also contains a high concentration of zinc, which is essential for a child's growth and development.

- Breastfeeding just after the birth also prompts your pituitary gland to release oxytocin, the hormone that causes the uterus to contract and expel the placenta soon after birth, helping to keep bleeding to a minimum.

- Studies show that breastfed babies have higher IQs than bottle-fed babies because of the essential fatty acids and other key nutrients in breast milk, despite the genetic makeup of the parents.

- A baby's digestive system is far from fully developed in the first few weeks, so the mother's milk is designed to meet its digestive and nutritional needs. As the baby and its needs develop, so does the mother's milk. Even when the baby's system is strong enough to accept solids, human milk is recommended as the main nutritional source until the baby is one year old. Human milk continues to boost the immune system for as long as it is offered. It takes between two and six years for a child's digestive system to reach full maturity (Ref. 5.1).

- Breast milk contains special proteins, antibodies, and white blood cells which help to protect the baby against infection and disease. Infant formulas don't contain such properties. As a result, bowel and lung infections tend to be more common in bottle-fed babies. Breastfeeding may also help prevent diarrhea and urinary-tract infections in babies. There is also evidence to show that the incidence of ear infections is significantly reduced in babies who breastfeed for longer than four months.

- It is nearly impossible for a baby to become allergic to its mother's milk.

- Breastfeeding may prevent milk- and other food-related allergies. There are more than 20 substances in cow's milk shown to be human allergens (Ref. 5.2). Colic and vomiting are often caused by cow's-milk allergy.

- Breastfeeding can help protect against allergies in babies in two ways. Firstly, breastfed babies are exposed to fewer allergens in the first months of life. Secondly, babies' immune systems are immature. They have previously relied on antibodies from their mothers while in the womb. Now that they are born, their systems are most suited to their mother's milk.

- Breast milk is convenient, cheap, and easy for most mothers.

- It is especially important for our baby to breastfeed for as long as possible if he or she is not being vaccinated, since breast milk helps to build the immune system and protect against disease.

breastfeeding disadvantages

There are very few disadvantages to breastfeeding.

• The only disadvantage that I found while breastfeeding my daughter Ella was that I had to be available at all times, which was fine until I needed to start working again. However, there are ways to cope with this.

• Some mothers may find it frustrating to watch what they eat for another few months after being "careful" for the last 40 weeks. Remember that it is not difficult to eat a good, varied diet, and it is important that you eat well for both your own and your baby's health.

• It is often hard to tell how much milk the baby is drinking from the breast, whereas the quantity of bottle milk can be regulated very easily. However, it is said to be impossible to over-feed a breastfed baby.

why organic breast is best

Organic breast milk is best. The longer a mother has been eating organically and reducing her exposure to environmental toxins, the better. Some studies have shown that pesticide residues and other harmful by-products of intensive farming can be passed to babies through breast milk.

In June 1999, this was documented in "Chemical Trespass," a World Wildlife Fund UK research report, which stated that babies were ingesting up to 42 times the World Health Organization (WHO) tolerable daily intake of dioxin-like compounds through breast milk.

disadvantages of cow's milk

Calves have different development and growth needs to that of human babies. Cow's milk is geared to meet a calf's needs. A calf's body grows extremely rapidly and doesn't have the need to develop a highly complex brain.

There is also a school of thought which maintains that pasteurizing cow's milk makes it difficult to digest and destroys useful enzymes (Ref. 5.3).

breast milk & nutrition

There are many advantages to eating a well-balanced diet. This is particularly true when breastfeeding. You will feel better, be more resistant to illness, and have more energy to cope with the new changes in your life.

However, for women who worry about the days they didn't eat as well as they could have, the following research should help put minds at rest.

The American National Academy of Sciences Subcommittee on Lactation confirmed in its 1991 summary "Nutrition During Lactation." "Women living under a wide variety of circumstances in the US and elsewhere are capable of fully nourishing their infants by breastfeeding them. Mothers are able to produce milk of sufficient quantity and quality to support growth and promote the health of infants—even when the mother's supply of nutrients and energy is limited."

Even with a less-than-ideal diet, a mother's milk is the perfect food for her baby. Studies conducted in developing nations indicate that even "mild malnutrition appears to have only a slight effect, if any, on milk output," and no effect on the composition of mother's milk. As Ruth Lawrence, MD, writes: "All over the world, women produce adequate and even abundant milk on very inadequate diets (*Ref. 5.4*)."

There are no complicated "diet rules" to follow and, contrary to popular belief, there are few foods that must be avoided by nursing mothers. If you are already eating a healthy diet, there is no reason to change while you are breastfeeding.

Most breastfeeding mothers find that they can eat what they like without their diets having any adverse effects on their babies. Occasionally, however—especially in families with a history of food allergy—a food in the mother's diet does affect her nursing baby. Some babies can be affected after their mothers have eaten something particularly strong or spicy, or when they have an unusually large amount of a particular food or drink.

foods to avoid

The most common offenders are foods such as chocolate, dairy products, wheat, and soy products. If the baby seems to be upset by a particular food or drink avoid it and continue breastfeeding —everything should be back to normal within a day or so. For more information about healthy eating guidelines, *see* pages 34–61.

The key to successful breastfeeding is plenty of rest, a varied diet of small, frequent meals, lots of water—drink at least 3 and a half pints a day—and getting gentle exercise.

breastfeeding
nutrition

the nutrients you need

...additional energy intake over and above pre-pregnancy intakes is needed during lactation.

As a guide to a healthy diet during the breastfeeding period, take a look at the recommended nutrients. For more information about the nutrients mentioned below, *see* pages 40–61.

Breastfeeding is an activity that demands energy. Even taking into account the fact that body fat stored during pregnancy is used to supply some of that energy, additional energy intake over and above pre-pregnancy intakes is needed during lactation.

As soon as weaning begins, a mother's energy needs start to return to her pre-pregnancy levels. For the purpose of setting estimated average requirements (EARs), breastfeeding mothers are classified in two groups. Group 1 mothers are those whose breast milk supplies all or most of the infant's food for the first three months only. Group 2 mothers are those who supply all or nearly all the infant's energy and nutrient needs for six months or more (*see* table below).

As soon as weaning begins, a mother's energy needs start to return to her pre-pregnancy levels.

stage of breastfeeding	additional EAR	
Up to one month	450 kcal/day	
1–2 months	530 kcal/day	
2–3 months	570 kcal/day	
	Group 1	**Group 2**
4–6 months	480 kcal/day	570 kcal/day
More than 6 months	240 kcal/day	550 kcal/day

protein

The normal reference nutrient intake (RNI) for protein is:

15- to 18-year olds: 45 g per day

19- to 50-year olds: 45 g per day

over 51: 46 g per day

These amounts increase for lactating women:

up to six months: an additional 11 g per day;

six months and over: an additional 8 g per day.

vitamin A (retinol)

The RNI for women is 600 mg per day, with an additional 350 mg per day for lactating women, totalling 950 mg per day.

vitamin B$_2$ (riboflavin)

The RNI for non-pregnant women is 1.1 mg per day, with an increase of 0.5 mg per day for lactating women, totalling 1.6 mg per day.

vitamin B$_{12}$ (cobalamin)

The RNI for non-pregnant women is 1.5 mg per day—a very small amount. Dietary deficiency is uncommon in the US. The RNI for pregnant women is women is 2.2 mg per day.

vitamin B$_3$ (niacin)

Lactating women need additional niacin to maintain adequate levels in breast milk over and above the increase that will occur as a result of increasing their energy intake.

vitamin C

The RNI for non-pregnant women is 60 mg per day. This increases to 80 mg per day during breastfeeding.

vitamin D

Vitamin D is obtained from sunlight. Lower levels of vitamin D have been found in placentas, so to avoid low levels in babies, it is recommended that pregnant and breastfeeding women should have a minimum of 10 mg of vitamin D every day.

calcium

The recommended calcium intake for women is 800 mg per day, with an increase to 1,250 mg for lactating women and 1, 350 mg for teenage lactating mothers.

magnesium

The RNI for magnesium is 280 mg per day for women. Lactating women need an extra 50 mg per day, totalling 330 mg per day. Teenage lactating mothers need an extra 30 mg per day.

zinc

The RNI dietary requirement for zinc for non-pregnant women is 15mg mg per day. This amount increases for lactating women:

0-4 months: plus 6 mg per day

over 4 months: plus.2.5 mg per day.

copper

The RNI for non-pregnant women is 1.5 to 3 mg per day, with an addition of 0.5 mg per day for lactating women, totalling 3.5 mg per day. Women who are pregnant are susceptible to excess blood levels of copper.

selenium

The RNI for non-pregnant women is 55 mg per day, with an extra 15 mg per day for lactating women, totalling 70 mg per day.

folate

The RNI for non-pregnant women is 180 ug per day, with an extra 60 ug per day for lactacting women.

"Eat when you're hungry" and "drink when you're thirsty" are the most important points to remember about nutrition and breastfeeding.

The international charity La Leche League International was formed over 40 years ago in the United States, and now has over 3,000 groups meeting in 62 countries. It provides information and support to any mother wishing to breastfeed.

It is a fabulous source of information and has put together many leaflets. "Common breastfeeding myths" is just one that is particularly impressive. Here are a few myths, taken from the leaflet, that La Leche League International can help to dispel. For further details about this charity and other breastfeeding support groups and counselors, see "Useful Addresses", page 143.

myth: If a baby isn't gaining weight, it may be due to the low quality of the mother's milk.
fact: Studies have shown that even malnourished women are able to produce milk of sufficient quality and quantity to support a growing infant. Most cases of low weight gain are related to insufficient milk intake or an underlying health problem in the baby (Ref. 5.5).
myth: Poor milk supply is usually caused by stress, fatigue, and/or inadequate fluids and food intake.
fact: The most common causes of milk supply problems are infrequent feedings and/or poor latch-on and positioning; both are usually due to inadequate information provided to the breastfeeding mother. Suckling problems on the infant's part can also adversely affect milk supply. Stress, fatigue, and malnutrition are rarely causes of milk-supply failure because the body has highly developed survival mechanisms to protect the baby during times of scarce food supply (Ref. 5.6).
myth: Some babies are allergic to their mother's milk.
fact: Human milk is the most natural and physiologic substance that a baby can ingest. If a baby shows sensitivities related to feedings, it is usually a foreign protein that has been "piggy-backed" into the mother's milk, and not the milk itself. This is usually handled by removing the offending food from the mother's diet (Ref. 5.7).

It is best that substances such as caffeine and chocolate, which contains theobromine, are consumed in moderation.

breastfeeding
myths

references

chapter 1

1.1   Old Testament, Judges 13, 3-4 &
Barnes, Bradley *Planning for a Healthy
Baby* (Vermilion 1994)

1.2   Stewart M. *Healthy Parents, Healthy
Baby.* London: Headline, 1995.

1.3   Wynn, A. and M. *"Prevention of
Handicap of Early Pregnancy Origin
Today—Building Tomorrow International
Conference on Physical Disabilities,"*
Montreal 4-6 June 1986; Antonov, A. N. J.
Pediatrics 30: 250-259 1974 *Children
born during the siege of Leningrad in
1942*; Smith, G. A. *J. Pediatrics* 30: 250-
259 1974 *"Effects of Maternal
Undernutrition Upon the New-born Infant in
Holland"*

1.4   Glenville, Marilyn PhD *Natural
Solutions to Infertility: How to Increase Your
Chances of Conceiving and Preventing
Miscarriage*
(Judy Piatkus Ltd. 2000)

1.5   Refior, Tiffany About.com.
www.vegetarian.about.com/food/vegetaria
n/library/weekly/aa011700a.htm

1.6   Brown, Judith E. *Nutrition and
Pregnancy: A Complete Guide from
Preconception to Postdelivery*
(NTC/Contemporary Publishing Company
November 1998)

1.7   Srivastava, K. C. et al *Danish
Medical Bulletin* vol 28 1981, pp 201-3
*"Prostaglandin E and 19-hydroxy-
prostaglandin E Content in the Semen of
Men with Normal Sperm Characteristics,
Men with Abnormal Sperm Characteristics,
Vasectomized, and Polyzoospermic Men"*

1.8   Davies, S. Zinc *1984-1985
Yearbook of Nutritional Medicine* pp. 113-
52 *"Nutrition and Health"* Bland, E. (ed)
(Keats Publishing, New Canaan,
Connecticut 1985)

1.9   *Preparation for Pregnancy*, Bradley,
Bennett, publ. Argyll Publishing 1997

1.10   Schwabe, J. W. R. and Rhodes, D.
Trends in Biochemical Science, vol 16
1991, pp 291-6 *"Beyond Zinc Fingers:
Steroid Hormone Receptors Have a Novel
Structure Motif for DNA Recognition"*

1.11   Hurley, L. S. *Physiological Reviews*
vol 61 1991 pp 249-95 *"Tratogenic
Aspects of Manganese, Zinc, and Copper
Nutrition"*

1.12   Krznjavi H. et al, *Selenium and
fertility in men, Trace Elements in Medicine*,
vol 9(2) 1992 pp 107-8.

1.13   Kumamoto Y. et al, *Clinical efficacy
of mecobalamin in treatment of
oligospermia*. Results of a double-blind
comparative clinical study, Alta Urological

Japonica, vol 34 (1988) pp 1109-32.

1.14   Jane Clarke's *Bodyfoods for life*,
publ. Seven Dials 1999 p.215

1.15   Fraga C. G. et al, *Ascorbic acid
protects against endogenous oxidative
DNA damage in human sperm*,
Proceedings of the National Academy of
Science, vol 88 (1991) pp 11003-6.

1.16   Dawson E. B. et al, *Effect of
ascorbic acid on male fertility*, Annals of
New York Academy of Science, vol 498
1987 pp 812-28.

1.17   Rushton D. H. et al, letter to Ferritin
and fertility, Lancet, vol 337 (1991) p 1554.

1.18   Jane Clarke *Bodyfoods for Life*,
publ. Seven Dials 1999

1.19   Bradley, Bennett, *Preparation for
Pregnancy*, Argyll 1997

1.20   Foresight Association
see Useful Addresses

1.21   Lodge Rees E., *"Trace Elements in
Health"* Editor, J. Rose, London,
Butterworths 1983

1.22   Bryce-Smith D. and Waldron H. A.,
*Lead pollution, disease, and behavior,
Community Health*, vol 6 1974
pp 168-75.

1.23 Needleman, Herbert L. et al. JAMA 1984 251 (22) and Lacranjan I, *Reproductive ability of workmen occupationally exposed to lead*, Arch Environ Health 1975 20

1.24 Rowland A. S. et al, *The effect of occupational exposure to mercury vapor on the fertility of female dental assistants, Occupational and Environmental Medicine*, vol 51(1) 1994, pp 28-34.

1.25 Bennett H. S. et al, *Breast and prostate in men who die of cirrhosis of the liver, American Journal of Clinical Pathology*, vol. 20 1950, pp 814-28.

1.26 Ellen Levine *Good Advice From Good Housekeeping*, www.homearts.com

1.27 Glenville, Marilyn *as before* (1.4)

1.28 Jick H. et al, *Relation between smoking and age of natural menopause, Lancet* vol 1 1977, pp 1354-5.

1.29 Stewart M. *as before* (1.2)

1.30 Himmelberger D. U. et al, *Cigarette smoking during pregnancy and the occurrence of spontaneous abortion and congenital abnormality, American Journal of Epidemiology*, vol. 108 1998 pp 470-79.

1.31 Barnes, Bradley *as before* (1.1)

chapter 2

2.1 Rice, R., '*Fish and healthy pregnancy: more than just a red herring, Professional Care of Mother and Baby,* vol. 6(6) (1996), pp. 171-3.

2.2 Reese, M.S. et al, '*Maternal and Parental Long-Chain Fatty Acids: Possible roles in preterm birth,*' *American Journal of Obstetrics and Gynecology*, vol. 176(4) (1997), pp. 907-14.

2.3 Wharton, 1992

2.4 Jameson, 1976

2.5 Doyle et al., 1990

2.6 Doyle et al., 1990

2.7 The US Institute of Medicine, report on Nutrition during Pregnancy 1990

2.8 Doyle, Wendy. *Healthy Eating for Pregnancy.* Hodder & Stoughton 1995 pp.35.

2.9 Department of Health (1992) *Folic Acid and the Prevention of Neural Tube Defects.*

2.10 Milunsky, A. et al., "*Multiviamin/folic acid supplementation in early pregnancy reduces the prevalence of neural tube defects*" JAMA 262:20, P2847-2852 Nov. 24, 1989.

2.11 Department of Health 1992 *Folic Acid and the Prevention of Neural Tube Defects.*

2.12 Rothman et al, New England *Journal of Medicine*, vol. 333(21) 1995, pp. 157-9.

chapter 3

3.1 Eisenberg, Murkoff,Hathaway, *What to Expect When You're Expecting*, publ. Simon & Schuster

3.2 Holford, Patrick *The Better Pregnancy Diet* Piatkus 1987

3.3 Holford, Patrick (*as before* 3.2)

3.4 Wynn A. & Wynn M., *The need for nutritional assessment in the treatment of the infertile patient*, J. Nutr. Med. 1: pp 315-324, 1990

3.5 BabyCenter, Inc www.babycenter.com

3.6 iVillage Inc., iVillage/ParentsPlace.com www.parentsplace.com

3.7 BabyCenter, Inc., www.babycentre.co.uk/general/4444html

3.8 Mother&Baby.co.uk, Emap Digital Limited,www.motherandbaby.co.uk

3.9 Holford, Patrick (*as before* 3.2)

3.10 BabyCenter, Inc., www.babycenter.com

3.11 Furuhashi, Nobuaki et al, *Effects of Caffeine Ingestion During Pregnancy, Gynecologic and Obstetric Investigation*, 1985, 19, 187-191

3.12 Infante-Rivard C., Fernandez A., Gauthier R., Rivard G. E., *Fetal loss*

associated with caffeine intake before and during pregnancy. Jnl.Am.Med.Ass. 270 (24): 2940-3, 1993

3.13 Stewart M., *as before* (1.2)

3.14 Mosher W. D. and Pratt W. F., *Reproductive impairment in married couples*. United States Vital and Health Statistics: National Survey of Family Growth, Series 23, No 11, 1987

3.15 Koller S, *Pisikofaktoren der Schwangerschaft*, Heidelberg:Springer-Verlag, 1983

chapter 5

5.1 American Academy of Pediatrics, *Policy Statement on Breastfeeding and the Use of Human Milk* (see Useful addresses)

5.2 Stigler U., *Preventive dietary management prenatal, neonatal, and in infancy*. Clin Ecol, 1985;3:1:50-54

5.3 H. and M. Diamond, *Fit for Life II: Living Health*, Bantam, London 1987

5.4 Ruth Lawrence MD

5.5 Nancy Mohrbacher 1997; 116-32; Wilde 1995, 401-6.

5.6 Dusdieker 1990, 737-40; Hill 1992, 605-13; Woolridge 1995; World Health Organization, 1995.

5.7 Hudson 1995, 886-92; Mohrbacher 1997, 97-99; Salmon 1994, 32-33

useful addresses

The American Academy of Pedriatrics
141 Northwest Point Blvd, Elk Grove Village, IL 60007-1098 USA
Tel 00 1 847 434 4000
Fax 00 1 847 434 8000

Foresight Association for the Promotion of Preconceptual Care
28 The Paddock, Godalming, Surrey, GU7 1XD United Kingdom
Tel 01483 427839
Fax 01483 427668

National Childbirth Trust (NCT)
Alexandra House, Oldham Terrace, Acton, London, W3 6NH United Kingdom
Tel 020 8992 8639
Fax 020 8992 5929

La Leche League (GB)
BM 1424, London, WC1 3XX United Kingdom
Tel 020 7242 1278

acknowledgements

For Jasmine Jade

So many people have provided information for this book that it would be impossible to thank them all. However, I must mention Becca and Emma at Mitchell Beazley for helping to turn my ideas into reality, and Phil, Miranda, and Bill for making the book look so gorgeous. A big thank you goes to James for his extensive research and for coping with the many late nights and weekends, Tanya for her nutrition advice, and Lizzie and Fiona for their assistance. And as always thank you to David, Pop, and Vicki for their continued support.

For everyone planning a family—hope this helps!

index